THE CHILD AND FAMILY

THE CHILD AND FAMILY

Contemporary Nursing Issues in
Child Health and Care

edited by
Bruce Lindsay
BA (Hons), RSCN, RGN, Cert Ed
Senior Lecturer in Child Care
Norfolk College of Nursing & Midwifery
Associate Lecturer
University of East Anglia, Norwich

Baillière Tindall
LONDON   PHILADELPHIA   TORONTO   TOKYO   SYDNEY

Baillière Tindall   24–28 Oval Road
W B Saunders   London NW1 7DX

The Curtis Centre
Independence Square West
Philadelphia, PA 19106–3399, USA

Harcourt Brace & Company
55 Horner Avenue
Toronto, Ontario M8Z 4X6, Canada

Harcourt Brace & Company, Australia
Limited
30–52 Smidmore Street
Marrickville, NSW 2204, Australia

Harcourt Brace & Company, Japan
Ichibancho Central Building, 22–1
Ichibancho
Chiyoda-ku, Tokyo 102, Japan

A catalogue record for this book is available from the British Library

ISBN–7020–1646–2

Typeset by Create Publishing Services Ltd, Bath, Avon
and printed in Great Britain by The University Printing House, Cambridge

CONTENTS

ACKNOWLEDGEMENTS

The publishers are grateful for permission to reproduce the following illustrations. To Stuart and Tracy Wise, Fig 2.1, Bruce Lindsay, Figs 3.1 and 3.3. To *Social Trends*, no. 22 (pages 43, 44, 46 and 47) for Figs 2.3a and b, and 2.4a and b. To Sam Lindsay for Fig. 3.2. To Jayne Taylor for Figs. 5.1, 11.1 and 11.2. To Sally and Richard Greenhill Photo Library for Figs 6.2, 7.1 and 10.1. To *Sweet, Mayes Midwifery*, 11th edn, Baillière Tindall, Table 14, for Fig. 8.1. To Baillière Tindall for Fig. 8.2.

CONTRIBUTORS

Theresa Atherton RGN, RSCN, DipN(Lond), Cert.Ed. *Lecturer in Child Care Nursing, Norfolk College of Nursing & Midwifery, Norfolk & Norwich Hospital, Brunswick Road, Norwich NR1 3SR*

Stephen John Happs MSc, BSc, RMN, RNMH, RNT. *Divisional Head, Anglia Polytechnic University, Chelmsford, Essex CM1 1LL*

Bruce Lindsay BA(Hons), RSCN, RGN, Cert.Ed. *Senior Lecturer in Child Care Nursing, Norfolk College of Nursing & Midwifery, Norfolk & Norwich Hospital, Brunswick Road, Norwich NR1 3SR*

Helen P Meehan BA(Hons), RGN, RM, ADM, Cert.Ed. *Midwifery Sister, Central Delivery Suite, Queen Elizabeth Hospital, Gayton Road, Kings Lynn, Norfolk PE30 4ET*

Terry Phillips Cert.Ed (Teaching), Cert.Ed (Youth Work), Adv. Dip.Ed (Language and Learning), (London) M.Phil. (UEA), Director of Courses for the Caring Professions, *Centre for Applied Research in Education, School of Education, University of East Anglia, Norwich NR4 7TJ*

Jayne Taylor BSc(Hons), RGN, RHV, DipN(Lond), RNT *Senior Lecturer, Suffolk College, Rope Walk, Ipswich, Suffolk, IP4 1LT*

Barbara Weller MSc, RSCN, RGN, RNT. *Independent Nurse Consultant, Lecturer, Chief Nurse Adviser, British Red Cross, Norfolk College of Nursing & Midwifery, Norfolk & Norwich Hospital, Brunswick Road, Norwich NR1 3SR*

Glenys Wise BA(Hons), RGN, NDN, PWT, DN (Lond), Cert.Ed, RNT. *Lecturer in Community Studies, Weavers Centre, Norfolk College of Nursing and Midwifery, Hellesdon Hospital, Drayton High Road, Norwich NR6 5BE*

FOREWORD

It is true to state thtat the society in which we live is currently undergoing rapid change. This has significant implications for the whole population including those engaged in nursing, and particularly children's nursing.

The title of the book is therefore particularly apt since it reflects a number of issues which are, at the present time topics of active debate. Much political rhetoric is being directed towards the virtue of family life. This does however raise the question of what is the family and can it be expected that the stereotyped image is still dominant. Within these questions and debates come other matters such as living in a multicultural society and the rights of children. These all have direct effects on the activities of those nursing who are engaged in working with children.

Nurse training has altered significantly within the past five years and much greater emphasis is now given to the sociological and psychological aspects of care. Although there are undoubtedly many books which include certain of the topics addressed, there has not been one as yet which seeks to interweave nursing and sociology in the same manner as presented here, and to discuss the unique role of the children's nurse. The possible future of children's nursing is also considered.

The book provides a refreshing approach to the subjects under consideration, and benefits from the contributions of experienced practitioners, whose knowledge and expertise can be disseminated through its pages.

Within each of the sections a wide range of topics have been considered and these have been linked to practical situations with which children's nurses have to contend on a daily basis, thus placing them in an appropriate perspective. Ethical problems which are increasingly matters of great concern to such people have received also appropriate attention.

It was a pleasure to be invited to write this Foreword, and thus to be associated, if only in a small way, with a book which has sought to fill a gap in nursing literature, by considering from a new perspective, topics which are usually discussed separately. The role of the family and its place in society is, however, central to children's nursing practice, and the subjects cannot be regarded separately.

The book should provide a valuable resource for all those engaged in the care of children since an innovative approach has been adopted, which will serve to enhance professional knowledge and understanding.

Pam Jefferies

PREFACE

The Child and Family is intended to be of interest to all people working in the health care of children. Primarily it is a book for children's nurses and students of children's nursing, but it is not a book *about* children's nursing. Instead the book collects together a series of contributions related to the health and nursing care of children. It does so with a number of intentions: to inform, to stimulate discussion, to suggest developments for practice and perhaps to generate controversy. And it does so because of the overriding belief that children deserve the best nursing care possible and that this nursing care cannot be achieved without an understanding of the context of children's lives outside as well as within health care settings.

The book is designed as a 'Reader' rather than as a comprehensive textbook. Taken in sequence the chapters move from a consideration of broad aspects of children in society through subjects of direct relevance to children's nursing to a closing chapter which proposes some possible ways of this field of nursing to move forward. This sequence is planned to give a 'wholeness' to the book but the chapters can be read singly, in any order or in any combination according to the needs or interests of the individual reader. Each section links together chapters with common themes but it would be equally valid for chapters to be combined in other ways to allow a particular interest to be considered or to enable comparison between the views of contributors.

The topics which are discussed are all, I believe, of importance to contemporary child care nursing. But because this is not a comprehensive textbook each reader will no doubt be able to identify further topics of importance which are not considered. Those which are here are those not normally considered in children's nursing texts, or are approached from a fresh perspective. They include subjects which have only recently come to be seen as valid areas of study for nurses, such as the effects of the media on development, and subjects which are often discussed in general nursing texts but which rarely receive such discussion in the context of children's nursing, such as nursing models. They also include areas of care which have long played a vital role in health care but which are only now being recognised widely as environments where child care nurses can be crucial participants, such as community nursing and the neonatal care unit.

The contributors to *The Child and Family* come from a variety of backgrounds. Three are child care nurses, but there is also representation from the fields of community nursing, health visiting, mental health and learning disabilities nursing, midwifery and general education. All share the belief that children deserve the best possible nursing care, but they were not asked to contribute because they all agree on what constitutes 'the best'. An advantage of multiple contributors is that they bring with them multiple perspectives on the subject matter. Agreeing that children deserve the best do not automatically lead to an agreement on what might be 'the best'. Indeed, while society and the environment continue to change it is highly unlikely that we will ever reach universal agreement on how to nurse children. In such a climate of change, constructive disagreement and discussion is vital to maintain the impetus for improvement: hopefully this book will help to carry forward this debate.

The Child and Family is the result of many hours of work by many people. My thanks go to my colleagues and friends who have contributed comments and suggestions, to Sarah James, my editor, and the staff of Baillière Tindall, and, of course, to my contributors. Most of all my thanks go to Julie, Sam and Alex for their support, encouragement and love through my many hours of absence from family life during the book's creation.

Bruce Lindsay
Milan
December, 1993

PART 1

THE CHILD IN SOCIETY

THE RIGHTS OF THE CHILD IN HEALTH CARE

Theresa M. Atherton
Norfolk College of Nursing & Midwifery

The phenomenon of human rights could be said to have its foundations in a fundamental belief in respect for the person. Affording and respecting those rights can be viewed as in-dicating the value that society places on the person as an individual or as a member of a group. As 'autonomous' adults we have it within our capacity to strive to have our rights respected as integral members of the society to which we be-long. Contemporary health care has reflected this change in attitude in that it now places the consumer at the centre of the delivery of care, as highlighted by the Patient's Charter (Depart-ment of Health, 1991a). The focus of this chapter is to explore the extent to which these values are reflected in the health care given to one of the most vulnerable groups within our society, namely children.

It might be expected that society has always placed a high value on its children, a natural consequence of a desire to see humanity carried forward into future generations. Sadly, though, this has not been the case. As recently as thirty years ago, the distress experienced by children was plainly and vividly seen within a health-care system charged with the task of care and protection.

Historical records and fictional literature of the time bear testimony to this fact, and possibly such experiences are within the memories of many people reading this chapter. Children admitted to hospital were separated from their families, visiting was restricted or prohibited, due to fears that families would bring infection into the hospital, cause unnecessary distress to the child and disrupt smooth running ward routines (Robertson and Robertson, 1989). Children were cared for in isolation from their families, the fundamental responsibility for protecting them during such a traumatic period of their young lives being denied. Fear, anxiety and feelings of abandonment, as natural sequelae to separation and developmental immaturity, failed to be recognised. Treatments, often causing pain and distress, were inflicted as a matter of course in the management of the disease, illness or injury. The long-term psychological consequences of such actions were not considered.

In acknowledging that the rights of children may have been abused in this way, it would be grossly unfair to lay the blame firmly on the doorstep of the health-care profession. The question of right or wrong in this case can only be seen in the light of evidence gathered in retrospect. Research on the effects of separation on the young child and studies of growth and development have allowed valuable insight into the world of the child. Evaluation in the light of knowledge and experience has enabled the care and welfare of children to be recognised as being essential within the value system of the health-care profession. Respect for the child as an individual with specific needs, and the fundamental right of each child to have those needs met, is now openly acknowledged. Perhaps, though, it would be wrong of us to dismiss our past as an embarrassing legacy. By the turn of the century, we may well be looking back and trying to understand how practices of today could have been allowed to happen. One can only practise within the limits of knowledge available at the time. Recognition of the past and hope for the future lead us to strive for the best possible standards of care for those children who become recipients of contemporary health care.

In today's 'enlightened era', no one would question that respecting the rights of children is implicit within a philosophy of family-centred care. The child-care nurse is now, more than ever, faced with the challenge of embarking on a therapeutic relationship with clients that must involve both the child and the family as equal partners. The potential imbalance of power between parties must be acknowledged, and every attempt made to minimise the risk of exploitation, particularly of the child, who may be the most vulnerable person in that relationship, and thus the most likely to be exploited.

Advocacy for both child and family is a key role for the child-care nurse. Within the therapeutic relationship, the nurse must ensure that individual rights are respected wherever possible. As a natural consequence, there is a predisposition for conflict between personally held beliefs and professional and legal responsibilities. In ensuring that a balance is achieved, and that due consideration is given to both child and family, the nurse must reflect on practice, basing actions on rational judgement through the ethical decision-making process, rather than on commonsensical knowledge, hunches or intuitions (Martin, 1989).

Family-centred care means a fundamental belief in the autonomy of the family in the care of a child (Charles-Edwards, 1991). Participation through negotiation is advocated at all levels of care. Under normal circumstances, this would not prove to be problematic when family, child and professional are in agreement as to what is deemed in the child's best interests. What poses a challenge and causes a conflict of interests is where there is discrepancy between the views of the nurse, child and family. It could be argued that the primary responsibility of the nurse is towards the child, but, in accepting this fact, the nurse might feel that the philosophy of family-centred care is being undermined, by interfering with the rights of the family to autonomy and self-determination. The personally held beliefs of the nurse may also come under threat as the very nature of the work undertaken by the child-care nurse of today precipitates involvement in such critical issues.

As a starting point, the intention is to expand the focus initially to investigate the more general context of how society perceives the rights of children and, perhaps more importantly, the way in which children perceive their own rights. In this way, the reader should be able to consider the significance of such provision within the context of health care. Let us begin by turning our attention to the concept of 'best interests'.

The Concept of Best Interests

Within our society, the family unit is held as being the means of providing a protective, supportive and loving environment within which children can be nurtured in order to develop to the fullest of their potential. Whatever the composition of that family, it is the stability of loving and caring adults that provides children with the essential requirements necessary for this to occur. The respect of children's rights can be seen to be implicit within this process, the family in the execution of its obligations being given the autonomy to decide what is both 'right' and 'good' for children. Adults are considered to have the ability through experience and maturity to make a rational choice as to what is deemed 'good' for a child. It is therefore natural to expect that the family will operate in the child's best interests.

If children are considered to be the sole responsibility of the family, then it could be argued that intervention by external authorities is unwarranted, but is it realistic to expect that all adults will operate to a common standard of best interests? As Mnookin and Szwed (1983) caution, what is deemed to be 'good' for a child is often a matter of subjective opinion. In situations where differing standards are being used, could there be a potential abuse of the rights of children, and if this is so, at what point should the decision to intervene become necessary, and to what degree? To intervene unnecessarily could be seen to be an invasion of privacy and an affront to a family's right to self-determination; to hesitate might be justifiably seen as negligence. Historically, there has been much criticism aimed at the way in which the state intervenes in the affairs of the family, as indicated by Geach and Szwed (1983), Stringer and Smith (1988) and Shapiro (1990). They argue that despite good intentions the consequences of such intervention have had disruptive and often damaging effects for children and their families.

Since the implementation of the 1989 Children Act (see also Department of Health, 1991b), the welfare of the child has assumed much greater significance. The legislation places the welfare of the child firmly in the forefront of any decision making by external authorities. Although no specific guidance is provided as to how the law should be interpreted, flexibility allows the best interests of the child to be respected whilst enabling professionals to intervene at times when the child is perceived to be in need. The Act stresses the importance of protecting children from what it terms 'significant harm', any decision made as to whether a child has, is or is likely to suffer significant harm being based on the perceived or actual threat to normal growth and development in comparison to that expected of a similar child.

Within the Act, the notion of family autonomy is seen as being of paramount importance. As the child's closest advocate, the family has a major part to play in decisions pertaining to the welfare of the child, and as such are given the freedom to exercise personal judgement as to what is deemed in the child's best interests. Assuming that the welfare of the child is protected, constraints imposed by society are limited, with intervention becoming necessary only where the child is considered to be at risk.

The Act also considers the wishes and feelings of children to be equally important, particularly in situations which affect them most directly. Where actions taken by the family are not considered to be in the best interests of the child and the welfare of the child is thought to be under threat, then society is responsible for intervening through the framework of the Act.

The question of who should have the right to decide what is in the best interests of the child is a particularly complex issue. Society has the duty to respect family autonomy whilst protecting the welfare of the child. Achieving a balance cannot be seen as being an easy task. It must be recognised that what, to the professional, constitutes acting in the child's best interests, might be very different from that perceived by the family. Professionals must exercise caution to ensure that personal interpretations of what constitutes best interests do not inadvertently prejudice families and children.

Recognising that differing standards of best interests are in operation perhaps leads us to question why this should be so. What are the influences that predispose to such differing perspectives? Perhaps the answer can be found within society itself.

How Society Perceives the Rights of Children

In attempting to explain the differing attitudes that influence society's approach to respecting the rights of children, Freeman (1983) describes three differing perspectives. His first theory is that of the 'child savers'. This theory acknowledges the vulnerability of children and thus favours a paternalistic approach, where children are perceived as being in need of protection. It legitimises the intervention of the state in child-rearing practices to ensure that the rights of children are uniformly protected. It places the decision-making function firmly in the hands of adults, the process being invoked by adults on behalf of children. Such policies as vaccination programmes and compulsory education could be viewed as being founded within this philosophy. The independence and status of children is not increased, neither is the provision of rights. The philosophy of the child savers engenders the belief that limitations are justifiably required in order that children are given equal opportunities, but it is adults who have the right to decide what is in the best interests of the child rather than the child themselves.

The second theory is that of the 'welfare rights' protagonists. This theory is not dissimilar to that of the child savers, but there is explicit acknowledgement of the good things that should be afforded to children. The United Nations Declaration of the

Rights of the Child (1959) could be seen as illustrating this philosophy, in that it emphasises the 'good' things that most people would subscribe to as wanting for their children, such as the right to adequate nutrition, housing, recreation and medical services. In assuming that children have the right to such provisions, then there is a moral duty and obligation placed on society to respect those rights through provision of adequate resources. In reality, this may prove to be an impossible task. How can there ever be an equality of resources for all children? If such resources cannot be provided, could children have a valid claim against a particular individual or society in general? Could parents and/or society be held morally accountable for a failure to ensure that those rights are respected? In the analysis of such a situation, the complexity of the relationship between rights, duties and responsibilities becomes clear. Freeman (1983) proposes that the declaration should be interpreted as a statement of obligation rather than of right, in that society can only offer to the child the best that it can provide.

The third theory is that of the 'child liberationalists'. Supporters of this theory would advocate that children be afforded equal rights with adults. Holt (cited by Freeman, 1983) suggests the following:

1   the right to equal treatment at the hands of the law;
2   the right to vote and take a full part in political affairs;
3   the right to be legally responsible for their lives and acts;
4   the right to work for money;
5   the right to privacy;
6   the right to financial independence and responsibility;
7   the right to direct and manage their education;
8   the right to travel, live away from home, choose or make their home;
9   the right to make and enter into quasi-familial relationships (i.e. to seek guardians other than parents);
10 the right to do, in general, what any adult may legally do.

The main thrust of this argument is the child's right to self-determination in that children should be allowed to decide on matters that affect them most directly. Acknowledgement is made that parents have a duty to nurture a dependent child, but the theory does not necessarily explain the consequences to the child in this situation. Freeman (1983) strongly criticises this approach as being 'politically naive and psychologically wrong', but he goes on to say that this theory makes us examine the age classifications for the involvement of children in the decision-making process. The cut-off points that are legally binding for such things as giving consent, getting married or buying alcoholic beverages could be considered within this context. The major difference between the child liberationalists and the child savers or welfare rights protagonists is that the former emphasise the protection of children's rights rather than the protection of children and take into account most emphatically the views of the child.

According to Freeman, there appears to be a continuum of perspectives. At one end, children are seen as vulnerable members of society in need of protection and at the other end as autonomous individuals with rights equal to those of adults. Perhaps our own personal belief system is influenced by the position we take along this continuum. This stance helps to determine not only the number and quality of rights to which we feel children are entitled, but also the extent to which we might strive to defend those rights.

But let us now focus on the position of the child. How much say does the child have in the way that rights are both determined and respected?

The Position of the Child in Determining Rights

From the child's perspective, claims will be made against individuals as a natural consequence of growing up. Such claims may vary in intensity from the toddler demanding to stay up late to an adolescent wanting to borrow the family car. Claims can be made against teachers, siblings, peer group and parents alike. Feinberg (cited by Freeman, 1983) calls these claims 'conscientious rights'. He continues by saying that although claims made in this way vary immensely in degree, all are relevant regardless of what the law might say.

Could it be said, then, that all such conscientious rights should be upheld as being true rights? Should all the demands that children make be respected in this way? Such a complex issue needs clarification.

Feinberg explores the relationship between claims and the establishment of true rights. He argues that the key to differentiating between a claim and a right lies in the ability of the child to justify that claim through reasoned argument. From this perspective, developmental maturity could be seen as being a crucial factor, the ability of the child to think in a rational manner being a necessary prerequisite for the translation of claim into right. If the claim is perceived as being both valid and relevant and proposed through a reasoned thinking process, then the likelihood of that claim being afforded the status of a right is increased.

The weakness of such a theory becomes apparent in a situation where the validity of a claim cannot be substantiated; for example, where a young child is unable to make a reasoned argument due to developmental immaturity. According to Feinberg, in this situation the claim of the child is still valid despite an inability to express that claim in an articulate way. But if the claim cannot be justified, how can the child stand a reasonable chance of being given a fair hearing? The answer to this question is difficult, but it must be acknowledged that it is almost certainly the family and/or society who have the power to decide to what extent such claims are respected.

Before progressing further, it might be beneficial for the reader to have a summary of the main issues covered so far.

Summary

1   Adults could be considered to be in the more powerful position when deciding what constitutes acting in the best interests of the child.
2   There can be no common understanding of what constitutes 'best interests', as any interpretation is a matter of subjective opinion.
3   Where differing standards are in operation, the rights of the child could be threatened.
4   Caution needs to be exercised when external authorities intervene in the affairs of the family. The Children Act (1989) provides a framework to guide such intervention.
5   The beliefs that adults have in respect of children's rights could be said to be influenced by the child-saver, welfare-rights or child-liberationist philosophies.
6   Children make claims against individuals and/or society, but it is likely that adults will decide whether there is a valid case for those claims being afforded the status of rights.

Respecting Rights within a Health-care Context

Having explored the background to the respect for children's rights within contemporary society, let us now investigate what all this has to do with the child-care nurse. Perhaps the starting point should be an exploration of the nature of the ethical decision-making process, as a means of understanding its significance within the context of health care.

The ethical decision-making process

The UKCC Code of Professional Conduct (1992) provides a framework to guide nursing practice. It focuses on the nurse's responsibilities and personal accountability for practice, and reflects the ethical considerations on which the whole ethos of nursing practice is based. Within the framework of the code, emphasis is placed on nurses examining the often complex motivations and the myriad of influences on those motivations, that contribute to the quality of care provided (Mahon, 1990). The concerns of the profession to set standards of care, and to monitor and evaluate that care, have meant that it is essential for nurses to examine their personal codes of behaviour in the light of professional practice. This process, called 'values clarification' (Brykczynska, 1989), involves clarification of personal values, beliefs and attitudes as a means of allowing insight into the complex area within which the ethical decision-making process occurs. But what is the nature of ethical decision making, and how does this differ from 'ordinary' decision making? In trying to answer this question let us attempt to define the term 'ethics'.

Ethics is a philosophical science involving the consideration of what ought to be, not necessarily what is. In considering what ought to be – that is, the 'ideal world' – a relationship with the so-called 'real world' can be explored. For the child-care nurse, this could be seen as attempting to achieve a balance between competing ideals: striving to respect human integrity and autonomy for both child and family on the one hand, whilst on the other, recognising and coping with the constraints of the health-care context. The so-called 'ethical dilemma' arises where there is not only a conflict of ideals but where there appears to be no clear indication as to what is the right or wrong decision from a series of alternative choices.

It might be true to say that the concept of an ethical dilemma is often associated with life and death issues focusing on complex and emotive issues, but perhaps this is to place too much importance on the sensational aspects of such cases. It must be realised that ethical dilemmas and the potential abuse of human rights are an inherent part of everyday life for the child-care nurse.

Making the best decision involves applying a rigorous and

analytical problem-solving process. All choices are examined to identify a course of action where the maximum 'good' and minimum 'harm' can be achieved for all those concerned. This can be seen to be the essence of effective ethical decision making. Models such as those proposed by Thompson and Thompson (1990) illustrate the stages of this process. Following such guidelines, though, does not necessarily guarantee that the best decision will in fact be reached, but as Thompson and Thompson (1990) state: 'intelligent, sensitive, caring individuals do make mistakes, but when they use a critical reasoning process, there is less chance for mistakes based on ignorance, personal biases, or strong paternalism'.

Ethical decision making relies on the ability of participants to make informal judgements as to what is deemed to be the best decision given a series of alternative choices. The soundness of such decisions could be said to be directly related to the level of moral reasoning being used. But how do we develop an ability to apply moral reasoning? Let us pause for a moment to explore the nature of moral development.

Moral development

The work of Lawrence Kohlberg (1984) is arguably the most influential in our understanding of the nature of moral development. He identifies three levels, each level being subdivided into two stages.

The first stage at level one, or the pre-conceptual level, suggests that the motivation for doing as we are told is based on the fear of punishment. Breaking the 'law' brings with it the risk of getting caught and being punished. Individuals balance such risks with the personal benefits of a particular course of action. An alternative perspective to the notion of punishment is that individual behaviour is motivated through the hope of achieving personal reward, or recognition – individuals wanting to be seen to be 'good'. Stage two of the pre-conceptual level is that of reciprocity. Doing unto others as we would have done unto ourselves could be seen as illustrating this principle.

The second, or conventional, level suggests that the individual's code of behaviour is modified according to the influences of society. Authority figures such as parents, religious leaders or teachers determine informal standards of what is or is not acceptable behaviour. Choices that the individual makes with regard to personal behaviour cannot be seen in isolation from the wider context of society's moral standards. The second stage of the conventional level relies on the adherence to more formal codes of behaviour such as those dictated by the police. The following of such rules and regulations is based on the fundamental belief that to do so is 'right'.

The third, or post-conventional, level of moral reasoning expands the notion of codes of behaviour to explore underlying principles. To follow a code of behaviour because it is considered to be 'right' predisposes to an either/or situation. There may be a need for modification of the code to ensure that the best decision is reached. Moral reasoning at this level requires highly developed cognitive skills in making what is considered to be an informed decision. The 'utilitarian' perspective of the greatest good for the greatest number could be said to illustrate this principle. The second stage of the post-conventional level is seen as encompassing a sense of 'duty' and the concern for 'justice'. The wider concerns of humanity are the major focus at this level.

Kohlberg's study of moral development could be summarised as expanding levels of concern. At level one, the primary focus is on the individual deciding on personal codes of behaviour. At level two, the focus is achieving congruence between personal codes of behaviour and those prescribed by significant groups in society. The third level, focusing on the wider concerns of humanity. Kohlberg does not imply that the development of morality is a linear progression from level one to level three. It is possible and expected that individuals will apply differing degrees of moral reasoning to differing situations, but it is recognised that the crucial factor influencing such functioning across the levels is an individual's stage of intellectual and cognitive development.

The nature of moral development can be seen as being influential in the ability of the child-care nurse to protect the welfare and rights of children within the context of ethical decision making. But what of the ability of the child and family to participate effectively? The ethical decision-making process relies on an equality of power between all participants to ensure that individual rights are respected.

The Balance of Power within Family-centred Care

Within a philosophy of family-centred care, it is expected that nurses will operate to the highest level of professional integrity when involved in decision making that affects both child and family. Although achieving an equality within the therapeutic relationship is seen as being fundamental to the practice of the child-care nurse, it must be recognised that there may be a natural imbalance of power distribution. When this occurs, there may be a risk of exploitation where the rights of both child and family are inadvertently compromised. So how and why should there be an imbalance of power? Let us analyse the differing perspectives of the decision makers.

The family

Not all illness in childhood results in a referral to the health-care services. Most is successfully managed by the family in the home environment. Assuming that the welfare of the child is not thought to be in danger, then few would question the right of the family to act in the best interests of the child. But where the disease, illness or injury is of such a severity that the family can no longer cope independently, then there may be little option but to seek professional help. The family having been swept into the system, their anxiety and stress precipitated by the child's illness may be compounded by feelings of inadequacy and unfamiliarity. This 'vulnerability' can naturally result in the family relinquishing control of their child to the 'expertise' of the professionals. How easy is it for the family to participate effectively when confronted with this situation? It would take a great deal of confidence to defend personal autonomy when confronted with the might of the 'competent' health service.

The child

The child is arguably most vulnerable during times of illness. Within the home environment the child relies on the care of a loving and supportive family in order to cope with any distress and anxiety. When the child becomes a recipient of the health-care system, this supportive environment becomes threatened. As previously illustrated, the family may relinquish control of the child to the 'experts'. Consequently, the child may no longer be able to rely on the family to care for and protect them. Developmental immaturity and a potential inability to express wishes and feelings to unfamiliar people only serves to compound an increasing sense of vulnerability.

The child-care nurse

At times when distressed families seek help, they do so because they do not have the necessary skills or knowledge to care for a child at home. In such a situation there is both implicit and explicit dependence on professional knowledge and expertise. Investment of such trust not only results in empowerment of the health-care professional but also inherently threatens the autonomy of the family. If knowledge is seen as being synonymous with power, and it is accepted that the child-care nurse is the person most involved in the daily care of the child and family, then it might be natural to assume that the nurse is in the more powerful position.

Achieving a balance of power

In accepting that vulnerability of the family is a natural consequence of a need to seek professional help, then it becomes necessary that it is both recognised and dealt with. Penticuff (1990) sees the empowerment of the family through the sharing of knowledge and information as producing equality and thus parity of power. Such exchanges could be seen to reduce the vulnerability felt, by placing the locus of control back in the hands of the family, thus facilitating their ability to participate effectively in any decision making regarding the child. But it must be acknowledged that distress and anxiety may interfere with their ability to become equal partners in the decision-making process. The child-care nurse must take this factor into account when ensuring that the welfare and rights of the family are respected.

But can an equality of power distribution be achieved so easily for the child? Due to developmental immaturity, children could be seen as being disadvantaged and 'powerless', and in such situations their wishes may be inadvertently overlooked because of an inability to express concerns in an articulate way. Distress and anxiety as a result of illness only serve to compound this fact. As we have previously discovered, the ability to participate effectively in ethical decision making depends on the participants' ability to make informed judgements, this ability relying on highly developed cognitive skills and moral reasoning. Allowing children to participate in the decision-making process would appear to be a potentially difficult task, in that it is relatively impossible to ascertain their ability to think in such a critical way (Alderson, 1991).

How then is it possible to know what the child feels regarding personal welfare? To what degree can we safely assume that the child is operating at a significantly high level of moral reasoning and cognitive ability to come to a decision as regards what constitutes their own best interests? Perhaps developmental theory can provide some clarification.

Piaget (1974), in his work on child development, proposed that the cognitive ability of the child could be directly related to age, children of certain ages being predictably expected to function at a particular level of thinking. But his work has been criticised, in that the proposed relationship between age and cognitive ability is too prescriptive. It is acknowledged that children develop through an orderly sequence of events, but because development may occur at different rates, age alone cannot be seen as being a reliable indicator of cognitive ability. It might therefore be natural to assume that reliance on the age of the child as a means of assessing an ability to make informed decisions is rather tenuous.

In this situation of uncertainty, achieving an equality of power within the decision-making process would appear to be particularly difficult. It is therefore essential for the child-care nurse to ensure that in respecting individual rights, the wishes and feelings of all participants are taken into equal account, so that children do not fall victim to the very system charged with the responsibility of protecting their welfare. As Brykczynska (1989) cautions:

> no one of the ethical agents should have a more important voice in the discussion just because of training, education or social class. All should be equal partners in the decision making, it will often be the child and family, if anyone, who carry the greatest responsibility overall, therefore great weight should be attributed to what they say, however 'unprofessionally' they say it.

As a means of exploring the complexities of achieving equality of power within the decision-making process, it is my intention to explore one of the fundamental concerns facing the child-care nurse during everyday interactions with children and families: the question of consent.

Children and Consent

Child-care nurses are involved in forming therapeutic relationships with both child and family. Following an assessment of need in which all parties have been involved, a plan of care is developed. The implementation of prescribed care to meet those identified needs is carried out within the philosophy of a family-centred approach, but may involve the nurse actively undertaking nursing intervention. This could involve administering medication, bathing the child, taking a temperature or encouraging the child to get out of bed following an operation. The question nurses must ask themselves is, how often do they seek the consent of the child before carrying out any prescribed intervention, and, possibly the most pertinent issue, what do they understand by the term 'consent'?

'Informed consent' is a term used where a person is both willing and able to agree to a course of action, based on full knowledge of what that action entails, and the likely consequences of that action. In her work on the ethics of using children in research, Lee (1991) explores the issue of consent. She examines three terms: 'consent', 'assent' and 'permission'.

She states that consent can only be given by an autonomous person who is able to control their own lives by being in a position of self-determination. Such a person would be able to decide whether to consent or not, based on critical analysis of the situation and the application of moral reasoning. This form of consent could be said to be 'informed'. It is debatable whether one could classify children as being autonomous individuals within this definition, as legally children are considered to be minors under the age of eighteen, and as such remain under parental control. It is also acknowledged that the degree of cognitive development necessary for the process of critical thinking and the application of moral reasoning is difficult to determine with any accuracy.

The second term is 'assent'. Based on the Piagetian theory of cognitive development, the child over the age of seven years might give agreement based on evidence of knowledge and understanding and a willingness to co-operate. The first criterion could be easily met; it is the second that might prove to be problematic. A child may listen to the explanation, show that they understand, but in the final analysis adamantly refuse to co-operate for a number of reasons – fear, pain or distress, to name but a few.

The third term is 'permission'. This is where the parent gives consent on behalf of the child. They are allowing their child to have the necessary intervention as it is perceived to be in the child's best interests. Lee sees permission being given for the child under the age of seven, where cognitively the child does not have the ability to fully comprehend the situation, or be in a position to apply moral reasoning in making a judgement as to which is the best choice given a series of alternatives.

Does Lee's explanation of the different degrees of consent help to guide the actions of child-care nurses in practice? In an ideal world, the answer would be 'yes', but the situation is far from clear when considering the complexities of caring for children. To illustrate the difficulties encountered, let us analyse an everyday situation of administering antibiotics to a child during the treatment of an infection.

It might be expected that a very young child would object profusely to the taste of the medicine, and refuse to take the prescribed dose. When faced with this situation, does the nurse ask for the consent of the child, explaining the need for the medicine? Would the child have the ability to understand that the medicine was necessary to treat the infection? According to developmental theory, the answer is probably 'no', and thus informal consent or gaining assent from the child would be inappropriate in this case. Options open to the nurse would be to ask the family to give the medication, administer the medication themselves, possibly against the will of the child, or to decline completely. In the situation of the nurse and/or family administering the medication, it could be argued that any attempt to restrain the child is in violation of the child's rights. To counter this accusation, it could be argued that the medication was being administered in the child's best interests and thus any anxiety and distress caused was justified. Not to administer the medication at all could also be viewed as not being in the best interests of the child, as the doctor in prescribing the medication has indicated that it is necessary for the treatment of the infection.

Let us now assume the child is of school age. According to developmental theory, the child is more likely to think in conceptual terms, in that the relationship between the illness and treatment is understood. It might be expected that, despite the taste, the child would understand the need to take the prescribed dose and thus comply with the request. In other words, assent is obtained. Informed consent could not be applicable in this case as the child is still considered to be a minor in the eyes of the law. The difficulty arises when, despite the child's apparent understanding of the situation, they refuse to take the medication. Should the nurse pursue the course of action disregarding the protests of the child, or should those protests be ignored, and what part should the family play in resolving the issue? The medication is necessary for the treatment of the infection, as indicated by the doctor. Assuming the family gives permission, then the nurse and/or the family is arguably obliged to administer the medication to the child. It can be seen that the balance of power rests firmly with the doctor, family and nurse. The child in this case appears to be the minority voice in the decision-making process. If the medication is administered against the child's wishes, have the rights of the child been abused? If the child appears able to understand the necessity for the medicine, and the consequences of refusal, it could be said that refusal to comply is the child's right. In practice, though, the health-care team would be professionally, ethically and morally bound to protect the welfare of the child and thus could justify the distress that might be caused. Permission of the family would be the only consent required in this situation. The child-care nurse, in administering the medication, would need to ensure that the child suffers the minimum amount of distress as a result of such action.

With the adolescent, who is developmentally able to understand fully the reasons for the medication and the consequences of refusal, the situation regarding consent is very different. Although children under the age of 18 years are considered by law to be minors, there is provision under the Children Act (1989) for children over the age of 16 years to give consent independently of both family and health-care professionals. If the child refuses the medication, and it is decided by the medical practitioner that the child is fully aware of the consequences of such a decision, then the law is flexible enough to allow the rights of the child to be respected regardless of the wishes of the family and/or health-care professionals. Where consent has been refused, the rights of the child should be respected.

The application of the different degrees of consent, as indicated by Lee (1991), can be seen to provide a framework for the child-care nurse during the execution of everyday nursing tasks involving children. The principles involved could apply to any situation of intervention, whether they be so-called routine tasks such as bathing the child, or taking a temperature, to more complex situations such as administering chemotherapy for malignancy, or assisting in the taking of blood specimens.

Conclusion

Respecting the rights of children within the context of contemporary health care has become a crucial issue for the child-care nurse. Achieving a balance between personal, professional and legal value systems relies on critical thinking and the application of high levels of moral reasoning, as well as recognition of the many factors that influence these processes. A balance of power must be achieved between child, family and professional to ensure that all parties are equally advantaged within the decision-making process.

With the implementation of the Children Act (1989) it has now, more than ever, become necessary for the profession to clarify the nature of the therapeutic relationship. Families and children seeking help from the health-care system do so at times of great stress and anxiety. Fear of the possible consequences of disease, injury or illness render them particularly vulnerable. This vulnerability automatically brings with it a dependence on those professionals perceived as having the knowledge and skills to alleviate distress and suffering. The child-care nurse must recognise this dependence and, within the framework of a family-centred philosophy of care, exercise caution to ensure that wherever possible the imbalance of power is not exploited and the rights of all concerned, particularly those of the child, are protected.

References

Alderson, P. (1991) 'Children's consent to surgery', *Paediatric Nursing*, Dec: 10.

Brykczynska, G. M. (1989) *Ethics in Paediatric Nursing*, London: Chapman & Hall.

Charles-Edwards, I. (1991) 'Who decides?' *Paediatric Nursing*, Dec: 6.

Department of Health (1991a) *The Patient's Charter*, London: HMSO.

Department of Health (1991b) *The Children Act 1989, an Introductory Guide for the NHS*, London: HMSO.

Freeman, M. D. A. (1983) 'The Concept of Children's Rights', in H. Geach and E. Szwed, *Providing Civil Justice for Children*, London: Edward Arnold.

Geach, H. and Szwed, E. (1983) *Providing Civil Justice for Children*, London: Edward Arnold.

Kohlberg, L. (1984) *The Psychology of Moral Development, Essays on Moral Development*, San Francisco: Harper & Row.

Lee, L. (1991) 'Ethical issues relating to research involving children', *Journal of Paediatric Oncology Nursing*, 8(1): 24.

Mahon, M. M. (1990) 'The nurse's role in treatment: decision making for the child with disabilities', *Issues in Law and Medicine*, 6(3): 247.

Martin, D. A. (1989) 'Nurses' involvement in ethical decision-making with severely ill newborns', *Issues in Comprehensive Pediatric Nursing*, 12(6): 463.

Mnookin, R. and Szwed, E. (1983) 'The Best Interests Syndrome and the Allocation of Power in Child Care', in H. Geach and E. Szwed, *Providing Civil Justice for Children*, London: Edward Arnold.

Penticuff, J. H. (1990) 'Ethics in pediatric nursing: advocacy and the child's determining self', *Issues in Comprehensive Pediatric Nursing*, 13(3): 221.

Piaget, J. (1974) *The Origins of Intelligence in Children*, New York: International University Press.

Robertson, J. and Robertson, J. (1989) *Separation and the Very Young*, London: Free Association Books.

Shapiro, R. (1990) 'Medical discrimination against children with disabilities: a report of the US Commission on Civil Rights', *Issues in Law and Medicine*, 6(3): 285.

Stringer, J. and Smith, P. (1988) *Family Courts – the Price is Right. Report for the Family Courts Campaign*, Family Courts Campaign.

Thompson, J. E. and Thompson, H. O. (1990) 'Ethics in theory and practice: applying the decision-making model – case study 1', *Neonatal Network*, 9(3): 75.

United Kingdom Central Council (1992) *Code of Professional Conduct for the Nurse, Midwife and Health Visitor*, 3rd edn, London: UKCC.

United Nations (1959) *Declaration of the Rights of the Child*.

2

THE CHANGING FAMILY

Glenys Wise
Norfolk College of Nursing & Midwifery

'The family is in decline.' Is there any truth in this statement? We bemoan the demise of the caring, sharing family, and yearn towards the model family presented to us by the media: the young, happy, well-heeled couple, a working father supporting mother at home with two clean, tidy and well-behaved children. But how true is this picture (see Figure 2.1)? Is the family in decline, or in the happy state depicted by the washing powder ads? I suspect the truth is quite different, and the reality lies somewhere in between.

The family as a unit has changed, and is continuing to change in response to social trends and attitudes and societal needs.

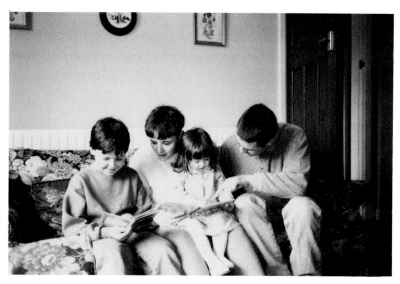

Figure 2.1   A typical family?

We are all part of at least one family: our *family of origin*, the family we were born into (also known as the family of orientation). We may as adults enter a second family, the *family of marriage* (also known as the family of procreation). This brings with it extensions of family networks, new family members and possibly new obligations. In the past, it was common for families to strengthen their ties and power by judicious marriages. In today's society, we feel we have free choice in whom we marry: this is an aspect to be considered later in the chapter.

The family is perhaps the strongest unit in society: Fletcher (1988) suggests that 'the family' lies at the very origins of society, and is one of the most basic groups for preserving social continuity. The early family, with its bonding ceremonies (marriage) and blood relationships, formed a strong group, able to identify itself by its 'clan' loyalties and obligations: society became based upon kinship and families, the regulating bodies, the agents of socialisation.

Closely bound up with the idea of family is the concept of marriage, or the legal binding together of an unrelated (or not closely related) man and woman. This new family, with the birth of children, will become a *nuclear family*. The nuclear family is not based on kinship (Harris, 1983) but on interrelated activities: the production of children does not depend on the formation of a domestic group; the interaction between the woman and man, whereby the man helps the woman to rear the children, is the group basis. Harris (1983) describes the nuclear family as having two sub-groups, man and woman, mother and children, with the man being the weak link. The existence of the nuclear family as a domestic group depends upon the relationship between the man and woman overlapping with the relationship between mother and children.

The nuclear family is said to be the ideal family for today's society, not bound by strong family ties, therefore able to move geographically to meet employment needs: supported by a welfare state at times of crisis. But the same facts are those used as criticism of the decline in family values! There is a myth which sees the extended family as 'the repository of all virtues and harmonies' (Segalen, 1986): the 'good old days', when large families all lived together, or at least in large communities, all cared for one another and rallied round in time of need. But it is perhaps as well to remember that the Poor Law was introduced as long ago as 1601 in order to provide for children, the elderly and handicapped persons whose families would not, or could not, care for them.

The Family: an Historical Perspective

Laslett and Wall (1972) dispute the general supposition that the domestic group of pre-industrial times was necessarily larger and more complex than that of today, and suggest that the term 'extended family' implies grandparents resident at all times: a highly improbable life expectation for many, particularly the peasant classes. Studies are presented (Laslett and Wall, 1972) which show that the mean household size remained constant at 4.75 from the early sixteenth century to the early twentieth century (the use of the term 'household' rather than 'family' holds wider connotations as it can include servants, or unrelated lodgers). It is therefore suggested that there is little evidence of the larger co-residential peasant family group giving way to the smaller nuclear family of today: the extended or co-residential family was *never* a common form of domestic group: in the nineteenth century only 5.8 per cent of households were shown to contain more than two generations (Laslett and Wall, 1972). What is not in dispute is the closer community residence of kin and affines (relations by marriage) of pre-industrial society. There was indeed no need to move; people stayed where their friends, family and work were: only in time of hardship were families uprooted any distance.

Industrialisation has, however, caused major changes in families, communities, society and societies (Segalen, 1986). The family has had to adapt and change, many of its functions have been taken over by the state or other organisations, but as a unit it still survives, its main function now being the rearing and socialisation of children. This latter function is now also shared with other organisations. Is the family losing all its functions? In fact, does it now have a function at all?

Despite the major upheavals, societal pressures and changes in marriage patterns, the family remains constant: a haven in a sometimes bewildering and threatening world. It is a refuge, and provides stability and support through good and bad times.

The popularity of marriage has not changed: there were 392,000 marriages in 1988, similar figures to 1961 and 1981 (*Social Trends*, 1992). However, of these marriages, in 1988 64 per cent were 'first' marriages, compared with 86 per cent in 1961: whereas remarriage, after the Divorce Reform Act (1969), has risen from 14 per cent in 1961 to 36 per cent in 1988.

Cohabitation, particularly in the 18–24 age group, has also increased greatly, from 4.5 per cent in 1979 to 12.4 per cent in

1988 (*Social Trends*, 1990), but cohabitation is usually before, rather than instead of marriage, and is often institutionalised by pregnancy – perhaps a conscious change of state?

Second or even subsequent marriages were not unknown in pre-industrial times: family patterns were in fact very unstable, due to high mortality (particularly maternal mortality) rates, and remarriage was common. Termination of marriage at an early age by death is relatively uncommon today, not as in the past. The death of children, too, was not uncommon and could have been no less painful than today, but these deaths were accepted as facts of life, to be endured. Segalen (1986) speculates on the effect on children of constant death and remarriage, and compares this with the attention paid to children involved in divorce today. The effects on children and their response was not considered important; basic survival was all that mattered. Children, particularly girls, might be sent away to domestic service at the age of 10–12, and might never see their parents again. The oldest child only could inherit, the others had to move on. Family patterns were in a constant state of transition. There was, even in earlier days, constant movement in the family network. The 'core' of the family remained the nuclear family, often with kin living in close proximity: but not the extended co-residential family, as is often taken for granted. Laslett and Wall (1972) note, in fact, that it is now recognised that the nuclear family predominates everywhere, even in the underdeveloped world.

So, if the nuclear family predominated in the pre-industrial era, and yet the Industrial Revolution was said to be the cause of the nuclear family group, has anything changed? Talcott Parsons, writing about the nuclear family in 1943, describes the effect of industrialisation:

> Industrialisation fragments the family, first by cutting it off from its kinship network, then by reducing the size of the domestic group to that of a small nuclear family which loses its productive, political and religious functions, and becomes simply a unit of residence and consumption. It shares its financial and educative functions with other institutions and its remaining function is to provide for the socialisation of children, and above all else, the psychological balance of adults. This domestic group, isolated from its kin, is based on a marriage between partners who have chosen each other freely, and its values are rational and pragmatic. Specialised male and female roles help maintain the existence of the family subsystem within the social system. The 'father's' role is 'instrumental' in that he provides the link

with society and material goods, and the 'mother's' expressive and exercised within the family.

(Parsons, 1943)

This was seen as being the 'ideal' family for an industrial society – social and geographical mobility made easier by the 'breaking' of family ties. Parsons' statement has been widely criticised: not least for its sexual stereotyping, but also for its functionalist approach in seeing the family as being moulded by the needs of society, rather than changing its structure to meet its own needs within a changing society. Nevertheless, there are elements of truth in there: but the 'breaking of family ties' has been disputed by many sociologists. Segalen (1986) reiterates that kinship relationships remained strong, even through the industrial nineteenth century, with 'family power' having an effect on industrial development. Families tended to work together, find jobs for its members, live in proximity. New or vacant jobs were 'kept' for relatives, particularly favourable jobs: this was true of both middle and working classes and often remains the same today, which is why areas of high unemployment tend to be in 'pockets'. Neighbours and relatives are relied upon for job information, rather than Job Centres.

The major industrialised companies, at the other end of the scale, were founded by, and kept within, wealthy families, with partnerships reinforced by marriage agreements; the basis of the communist ideology of the family being the 'cornerstone of capitalism' which resulted initially in the abolition of the family unit following the 1917 revolution: a decision reversed a few years later when the birth rate plummeted, and vandalism and violence escalated. 'The family' was reinstated as an agent of moderating social control.

There have thus been changes in family structure, with the 'core' family (the nuclear family) remaining the main unit in the past with kin and affines living within the close community and relying on one another in times of crisis. Today's family is still the nuclear family, but there have been other changes, related to living conditions and expectations rather than controlled by social needs.

The Family: Changing Structure and Expectations

Generally families no longer live in the close proximity of yesteryear, but contact is still maintained, and ties reaffirmed at family occasions (christenings, marriages, funerals). Individuals

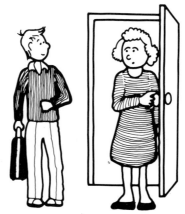

My mum's second cousin Doris is your husband's grandad's niece

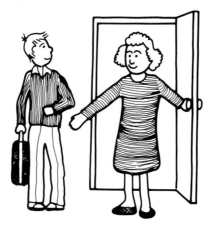

Oh you're family! Come in!

Figure 2.2

regard themselves as part of the larger family networks, not just a member of a nuclear family. Kinship is still important, it gives a sense of belonging and a system of identification: it offers an introduction into 'new' family networks and ensures acceptance even amongst previously unmet kin. Kinship implies a social (not necessarily biological) relationship, with rights, duties and obligations. Marriage creates new sets of kin, therefore it is the creation of group relationships as well as individual partnership. This brings us back to the concept of free choice of marriage partner, with the notion of romantic love underpinning the whole. Harris (1983) points out that in no society are groups entirely uninterested in their child's choice of mate: they will be gaining a new set of kin. Parents will live in the kind of area, mix with the kind of people, send their children to the kind of school, use the kind of leisure facilities of the type of group they would like their children to marry into. Manipulation of marriage choice is covert, but firmly in position.

Marriage, as stated previously, is not going out of fashion. What are changing, and fairly rapidly, are three main aspects of family life: increase in divorce, births outside marriage, and the changing role and expectations of women.

First, *divorce* was seen until relatively recently as personal failure, instability or the punishment of a partner at fault; now divorce is commonplace. The dramatic rise in the eighties has continued: nearly four in ten (37 per cent) of marriages now end in divorce (*Guardian*, 9 July 1991). This is reflected in the rise in lone (divorced) mothers from 24 per cent of all marriages in 1971 to 44 per cent in 1987 (*Social Trends*, 1990). Numbers of single (unmarried) mothers have also risen, from 16 per cent in 1971 to 29 per cent in 1987 (*Social Trends*, 1990); but lone (widowed) mothers have dropped from 31 per cent to 8 per cent over the same period.

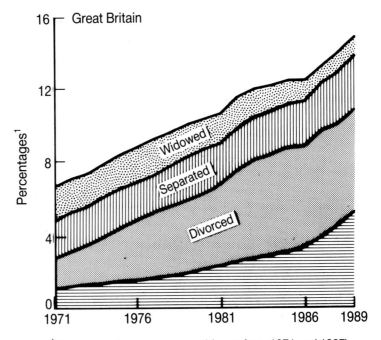

[1] 3-year moving averages used (apart from 1971 and 1987).

Source: Office of Population Censuses and Surveys

Figure 2.3a   Proportion of all families with dependent children headed by lone mothers: by marital status

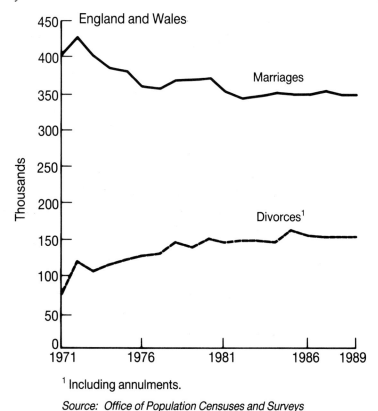

[1] Including annulments.

Source: Office of Population Censuses and Surveys

Figure 2.3b   Marriages and divorces

Serial monogamy in the past was due to high maternal mortality: nowadays couples can expect fifty or more years together, so is divorce really so surprising? The fact which has become apparent in recent years is the increasingly earlier age at which marriages are dissolved. Segalen (1986) examines this fact, and suggests that the characteristic identifying this group is social and professional: it is mainly the middle-class group who find divorce financially and culturally more acceptable and accessible. Segalen suggests that younger women in this group are more likely to have educational and/or professional qualifications and are therefore able to be independent. Divorce is not as common amongst the working class. Here marriage is a means of legitimising the *status quo*, and divorce is slow and expensive. The upper classes also tend not to divorce, it is not compatible with the transmission and maintenance of social, economic and cultural capital (Segalen, 1986).

The main increase in divorce was seen after the Divorce Reform Act 1969, but Fletcher (1988) suggests that most of these

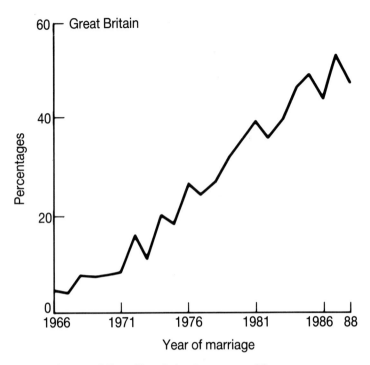

Source: *Office of Population Censuses and Surveys*

Figure 2.4a   Proportion of women who cohabited with their future husband before marriage: by year of marriage

marriages had already broken up; the Act allowed legitimisation of an existing state, and regularisation of an already established alternative stable union. He also suggests that the higher divorce rate might be reflective of higher expectations of marriage. Divorce cannot be seen as a rejection of marriage, or the family, as it is often followed by remarriage.

Secondly, *births outside marriage* have risen sharply over the last thirty years, and by 1990 were 28 per cent of all births, compared with 12 per cent in 1980 (*Social Trends*, 1992). Two-thirds of these children were born to women under 25. There has been an increase in the proportion of births outside marriage being registered by both parents, from one in twenty-five in 1971 to one in five in 1990, and of these 71 per cent gave the same address, indicating a stable non-marital relationship (*Social Trends*, 1992). Illegitimacy no longer carries the social stigma of years gone by, and the Family Law Reform Act 1987 abolished all legal discrimination against such children. The father, however, does not have the legal right to be the child's

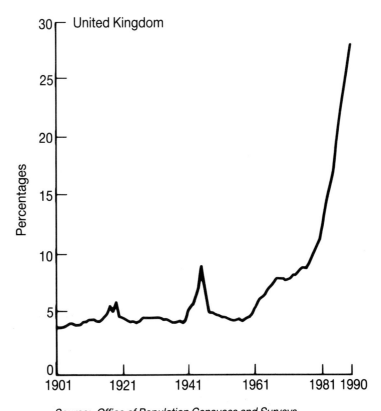

Source: *Office of Population Censuses and Surveys*

Figure 2.4b Live births outside marriage as a percentage of all births (Great Britain)

guardian unless he adopts the child, or marries the child's mother.

In the past, children offered for adoption were usually those born to single mothers (the mother being 'persuaded' to give up the child for her 'own good'), or the children of broken marriages (before the 1975 Children Act), when the courts thought it was 'best' for the child to be in a two-parent family. Adoptions have fallen considerably from 22,500 in 1974 to 7,300 in 1988 (*Social Trends*, 1990).

Thirdly, there have been *changes in the role and expectations of women*, more than those of men, over the last century. Two world wars involved a dependence on women for labour, leading to a realisation for many women of their economic independence, sadly often lost after the war. Women have increasingly become part of the labour market in the last thirty years, and together with improved equity in education and

qualifications, this led to higher expectations. Life expectancy
has increased, and the introduction of the contraceptive pill in
the 1960s gave women control over their own fertility. Women
are now likely to have fewer children, earlier in the marriage.
Child-bearing trends suggest a growing tendency to remain
childless: it is expected that 17 per cent of women born in 1955
will not have children, compared with 10 per cent of those born
in 1945 (*Social Trends*, 1990) or to have only one child: now 10
per cent of all families, compared with 2 per cent in 1980 (European Commission Survey, 1991, reported in the *Guardian*.)

The proportion of women bearing four children fell from 20
per cent of those born in 1930–35 to 12 per cent of those born
in 1945, and a further fall is predicted. The average number of
children per family fell between 1971 and 1981 to 1.8 and has
remained constant since then. The average career break for
women having children is now 2.4 years as contrasted with 6
years in the 1960s. Although the modern mother may go to
work, she is still expected to undertake the traditional 'housewife' role once she gets home. The sexual division of labour may
be blurring, but it is still sharp and clear at the edges. It is interesting to note that the 'acceptable' professions for women are
those which appear to be an extension of the 'mothering' role,
such as nursing, teaching and social work.

To sum up the changes in family life over the last 100 years:
the nuclear family remains intact, but with many of its functions
lost; the 'extended family' is used in a looser connotation to
mean kin with whom one integrates relatively closely; family
networks remain strong but looser; they have also become
wider through divorce and remarriage. Changes in social attitudes mean that more children are born outside marriage; more
marriages end in divorce; and more women are economically
independent inside and outside marriage.

Today's Family: Parents and Children

What does all this mean to the children of the family? Fletcher
(1988) describes the modern family as:

1 Founded at a relatively early age of husband and wife, and
   with increasing longevity, therefore of long duration.
2 Consciously planned to limit the number of children.
3 Therefore small in size. Typically husband, wife and two
   children.
4 Separately housed (satisfying a desire for independence and

privacy) and usually in a material and neighbourhood environment much improved on those of earlier periods.

5 Economically self-responsible, self-providing and therefore (a) relatively independent of wider kin and (b) living at a 'distance' from them – frequently geographic, but also in terms of a diminished degree of intimately shared social life.

6 Founded and maintained on a completely voluntary basis by partners of equal status: entailing therefore a marital relationship based on mutuality and consideration and sharing of tastes, seeking to be a 'marriage of true friends'.

7 Democratically managed in that husband and wife (and frequently children) discuss family affairs together during the taking of decisions.

8 So centrally concerned with the upbringing of children as to be frequently called 'child-centred'.

9 Widely recognised by government and the whole range of social services as being crucially important for the life of individuals and society alike, and helped in its efforts to achieve health, security and stability by a wide ranging network of public provisions.

To take Fletcher's eighth statement, this child-centredness is now often seen as the main function of the family: it even echoes Parsons' disputed quotation (see page 25) that the family's 'remaining function is to provide for the socialisation of children'. The loss of functions such as the political, productive, recreational, educational and religious, together with the establishment of the smaller, more independent family unit, has come to mean concentration on the one aspect of production and creativity left to the family – children. The child within the family, therefore, has tended to take on a new significance: the family is judged by its 'child production'. Children are seen not only as a continuation of the family identity (Harris, 1983) but also as a proof of their social worth, by their achievements and social graces.

The status of children in society has changed considerably over the last century: the child in Victorian times was the means of continuing the family and supplementing income. Children as young as four years of age were taken into factories, or expected to work on the land. Child mortality was high, and for children to be seen as individuals was a luxury: the child was seen as a contributing family member.

The idea that very large families were the norm before contraception was available is not totally correct: the numbers of births were controlled by several factors, not least infant and maternal mortality (Harris, 1983), plus economic conditions, and poor diet could have affected fertility or caused miscarriage. The average number of children per family in the nineteenth century was four (Harris, 1983), of whom only two would reach child-bearing age. The accepted way of life was a high birth and high death rate. Children were part of the whole community, socialised by parents and grandparents, educated by older siblings, farmhands, servants: a collective rather than an individual responsibility.

Attitudes to children began to change as a result of two factors: first, the drop in infant and child mortality around the turn of the century. There was more likelihood of the child surviving to adulthood, and the child as an individual came to be seen as irreplaceable (Oakley, 1976). Family size then began to be controlled as parents felt surer of the survival of their children: they began to want to ensure the future of the *child* rather than the future of the *family*. This was a deliberate decision by parents, rather than random 'natural selection', and with it came a new attitude to children and childhood.

Secondly, the period of childhood lengthened as education became compulsory, and the child remained dependent on the adult until adolescence, rather than 'earning his keep' from as early an age as possible.

Socialisation of Children: Whose Responsibility?

The family grew smaller and more private, and the children became more valued. The move was to have fewer children, but for them to be healthier and better educated. As a result, both education and medicine have assumed increasing importance, and have taken over many of the functions of preparing the child for adulthood.

Increasingly children became separated from their parents during the day, during which time their socialisation agencies were either peer groups or unrelated adults (teachers), whose norms and values might well be very different from those of the family.

The 1950s brought the development of a more permissive type of upbringing, with paediatricians and child psychologists maintaining that too close a dependence could harm character development and the child's need to discover autonomy (Segalen, 1986). There were conflicting ideas on the need for maternal presence, particularly for the young child. Women were torn between psychologists telling them that the mother–child relationship is all-important, and social and feminist values stressing the importance of self-fulfilment in work. Reconciliation of these conflicting views caused guilt feelings and anxiety.

The family is still the main agent of primary socialisation: Fletcher (1988) describes the family as 'the avenue' through which the child is introduced to wider social groupings – through kin, neighbourhood and, eventually, society.

Children from the ages of 3–4 years will have increasing contact with others in the same age band, through nursery schools and playgroups, then in primary school. Peer groups are described by Giddens (1990) as friendship groups of children of a similar age. Traditional societies formalise these groups into age grades, the whole group moving through the responsibilities and rights of their age band together, not as individuals. Western society also tends to age-band children without the conscious realisation of this: children spend most of their time with their peers, and it is within this group that the child explores rules of conduct and behaviour. Parents are needed to help the child towards autonomy, and to cope with anxiety and change.

The adolescent belongs strongly to the peer group, and wishing to become totally non-conformist, becomes ultimately conformist with the group. This is a time of possible family conflict, but the rebellions are often against society's rules rather than those of their family.

'Childhood' has become a distinct part of life: the stage between infancy and adolescence. The recognition of childhood, the period of education, is a relatively recent one: as is the idea that children have rights, and that child labour is unacceptable (Giddens, 1990). Until the twentieth century, children moved from a lengthy infancy into a working life, and for many children in Third World countries this is still the case.

Relationships between parent and child have also changed from strictness to quasi-friendship. The Newsons (quoted in Harris, 1983), in their longitudinal study (1963, 1968, 1976) found that their respondents noted a change in their own and their children's childhoods, in affectivity and psychological closeness. They noted a greater openness between parents and children, with more shared interests. This was related to smaller family size and better living conditions. But this greater freedom could also lead to greater tension: the child could, by certain actions, upset the whole household, but might be unable to comprehend the possible result of the actions.

The Newsons reported that, for a surprising 75 per cent of the sample, being 'struck with an object' was a likely occurrence. Resolving conflicts by force or threat of force caused conflict for parents: a tension between a desire for closeness, friendship and the need to control unacceptable behaviour.

Parent–child interaction is seen by the Newsons as rooted in conflict, bargaining supported by threats. The desire to see the child as a 'friend' appears to require an adult response from an immature, not fully socialised person who may not be capable of making the correct response. Society seems once again to be reducing the period of childhood, by expecting children to behave as adults. Children are exposed to adult entertainment such as television pictures of violence, murder and catastrophes, as well as the addictive soap operas offering some very peculiar human behaviours, from an early age: children are rarely portrayed by the media as 'normal' children but as small adults. Children who respond in what they perceive as an adult fashion, which may be totally inappropriate, may find themselves, confusingly, punished.

To be a parent nowadays is difficult: the parent is held socially responsible for the character and behaviour of the child. The child's behaviour is seen as a measure of the moral and personal worth of the parents: this implies that the power of the child is enormous, and can be used to diminish parental control. But if parenthood is a dilemma for parents, so must childhood be for children (Harris, 1983). The child is rendered dependent, yet expected to be independent; treated as a friend, a small adult, yet rebuked if it seems to be an adult response that is given; shown the world of adults via the media, but punished if the behaviour is copied.

There is also what Giddens (1990) refers to as the dark side of the family: activities which belie the rosy media image of family warmth and security, the worst of which can only be sexual and physical abuse of children. Until relatively recently it had been assumed that strong taboos meant this behaviour was rare, but recent attention by welfare organisations has found it to be widespread, and mostly within the family. Sexual abuse is commonly between fathers or stepfathers and young daughters, and is described as an exploitation phenomenon, often with force or threat of violence involved. Children are dependent within the family, and vulnerable to parental demands and pressures.

However, violence and abuse are not only carried out by parents against children: disturbing evidence has been documented (*The Independent*, 23 July and 19 August 1992) of parents attacked by children, and of sibling violence. 'Childline' is reported as receiving 15 per cent of its calls from abused or bullied siblings. The same report documents two murders and thirty cases of grievous bodily harm between siblings during 1991 on file at Scotland Yard.

Is this a new phenomenon? Or are we belatedly recognising an underlying thread which has remained hidden until now? It would be easy to lay the blame on the intensification of stresses within the smaller nuclear family, but this is surely a simplification, and overlooks the complex and rapid changes in society as a whole. The family, and the children within it, have been and continue to be subject to major stresses and conflicts from both within and outside the boundaries of the group. Change in both structure and function have resulted, but not in a societal and cultural belief in the family as a desirable group.

Families, despite their similarities, are composed of individuals, of whom the adults will have negotiated a relationship in which they feel comfortable: children do not have this advantage. The decision of the domestic group to live together implies a closeness, and dependence upon one another. Identification of the individual's role within the family becomes the focus of their personal life, and the concept of 'family' has now become almost interchangeable with the concept of 'home' (Oakley, 1976), reinforcing the boundaries of the group.

The Child in a Health Dependency Situation

The child in a health dependency situation needs to remain within the domestic grouping if at all possible. To take the 'family'-equals-'home' analogy, this is where the family is, this is where the child should be. Health-care professionals should be going to the child rather than vice versa.

If the health dependency situation warrants hospital admission of the child, then the family should be taken into partnership of care. The nuclear family can be viewed as an interdependent organic unit, each part interacting with the other to form a whole. As such, the child should be seen as part of the whole, with the other parts/members essential for the child's continued well-being. Continuation of the system which signifies normality for the group, and the individuals within it, should be maintained and actively encouraged. Normality of everyday life brings sense and stability when the situation is abnormal. Removal of one group member from the whole has a greater diminishing effect on all members than might be expected or apparent.

The child is not a separate entity, to be considered in isolation. The child's main need (which may not be the most urgent health-care need) is to be within the context of family membership. This is normality, this is the most health-effective, socially effective, psychologically effective and probably cost-effective context within which to treat dependency situations.

Families should be encouraged not only to be partners in care, but also to take prime responsibility for their child in the meeting of needs, with help and support when needed, both in the immediate caring situation and also in ensuring that domestic worries or concerns are not an obstacle.

Families of so-called 'primitive' societies move into hospital with their child, continuing everyday normality, nurses and doctors giving the specialist and technical treatments necessary. A picture comes to mind from a recent TV programme (*Stories from an African Hospital*, Channel 4, 1991) about an abandoned boy admitted to hospital in West Africa who was regularly asked by other parents 'Who is with you?', 'Who is looking after you?' as this aspect of care was not seen as the nurse's role. Child care in hospital in industrialised countries, particularly the United Kingdom, has come a long way from the time when parents were barred from seeing their child in hospital, to prevent 'upsetting the child', but the continued emphasis on the medicalisation and professionalisation of child care cannot be truly seen to be in the child's best interests, and the effect is to marginalise the parents, rendering them powerless in a situation in which they should be in control. Perhaps there are lessons to be relearned here.

Children cannot be seen as separate from their families. Family ties and commitments are no less strong then they have ever been. We have seen the narrowing of family obligations and functions to centre upon the child, whose survival and wellbeing *as an individual* has become the *raison d'être* for the parents. The child has moved from being the collective responsibility, and possible continuance of the family of Victorian times, to being an integral family member of the smaller, more independent nuclear family of today: an important, valued individual essential to the 'wholeness' of the group.

The family as a unit remains the key group within society: its size, shape, structure and functions may have changed dramatically, but each member within the unit recognises a social and emotional interdependence enabling the whole group to remain healthy, in the widest context.

Family decline? No. Family change? Yes; and change is always threatening, particularly when it appears to undermine strongly held values and beliefs. Fletcher (1988) describes the emergence of three main perspectives in recent years. The first sees the 'new libertarian values' as responsible for all ills in society; the deterioration of family life, increase in separation and divorce, single parents living in poverty, unsatisfactory step-parents, children abandoned, illegitimacy, child abuse – all these are laid at the 'deteriorating family's' door.

The second perspective blames the small nuclear family unit for its obstinate hold in a changing world: it is the problem, causing mental stress, disorder, outbreaks of violent rebellion, deprived families seen as failures. The 'tyranny of the family' is held to blame here.

These two perspectives tend to be those which 'grab the headlines' and are strongly held by some people, but Fletcher describes a third view, that something is not quite right, but do we have to blame the family? This view recognises the changes within the family, particularly since World War II: improved living conditions; the improved status of women and children leading to improved family relationships; the provision of a welfare state and National Health Service means theoretically that no one should be hungry, homeless or unable to obtain treatment for illness. These are improvements, changes that society wanted, but the social problems are still there. Has the family in some way been undermined, or are the problems more symptomatic of rapid societal change?

What emerges very clearly is the continuing strength and importance of the family, and of its members to one another. The child is not divisible from the family, whatever its individual structure may be.

The concept of the two-parent, two-child family as the norm is a myth, and probably always has been a myth; nevertheless, it is this mythical family that is used as the basis for policy making, and that tends to be the family structure of expectation. Families come in all shapes and sizes, and it is the 'whole' that is important, rather than the sum of the parts.

References

Childline Report, information from *The Independent*, 19 August 1992, 'Is there a little monster in your house?', p. 14.

Fletcher, R. (1988) *The Shaking of the Foundations: Family and Society*, London: Routledge and Kegan Paul.

Giddens, A. (1990) *Sociology*, Cambridge: Polity Press.

Guardian, 9 July, 1991 'Mixed Doubles', p. 1.

Guardian, 29 July, 1991 'More parents opt for one child', p. 4.

Harris, C. C. (1983) *The Family and Industrial Society*, Boston: Allen and Unwin.

Laslett, P. and Wall, R. (1972) *Household and Family in Past Time*, Cambridge: Cambridge University Press.

Newson, J. and Newson, E. (1983) 'Longitudinal studies' in C. C. Harris, *The Family and Industrial Society*, Boston: Allen and Unwin.

Oakley, A. (1976) *Housewife*, Harmondsworth: Penguin.

Oakley, A. (1981) *Subject Women*, Harmondsworth: Penguin.

Parsons, T. (1943) 'The kinship system of the contemporary United States', *American Anthropologist*, 45.

Segalen, M. (1986) *Historical Anthropology of the Family*, Cambridge: Cambridge University Press.

Social Trends (1990), No. 20 London: HMSO.

Social Trends (1992), No. 22 London: HMSO.

Stories from an African Hospital, Channel 4, 1991.

Additional Bibliography

Anderson, M. (1980) (ed.) *Sociology of the Family*, Harmondsworth: Penguin.

Bott, E. (1963) *Family and Social Network*, London: Tavistock.

Helman, C. G. (1990) *Culture, Health and Illness*, 2nd edn., London: Wright.

3

INFLUENCING DEVELOPMENT: THE MEDIA

Bruce Lindsay
Norfolk College of Nursing & Midwifery

A child's environment forms a rich source of developmental influences. From early contact with the immediate family through experiences with other family members, neighbours and friends to contact with the wider community, each child interrelates with many individuals and groups. The child's home, neighbourhood and schools offer varied examples of how people work in competition or co-operation, of success and failure. Occasional experiences – for example, of hospitals or of nurses – may well serve to influence for life the development of a child's understanding of concepts such as health care or health carers.

Television is one such environmental influence. A rarity forty years ago, it is now almost universally accessible to children in the Western world. With its older relatives such as radio and magazines and its younger sibling the video-recorder, television is part of the communications media. These media exert a strong and lifelong influence on the development of children in the late twentieth century. Their role in children's lives is now so important that we must attempt to understand it in order better to understand the children themselves.

Children and the Mass Media: Assessing the Influence

Do the mass media influence children and adolescents? The short answer must be 'yes' even if it's based simply on an informal assessment of the amount of output aimed solely or predominantly at the under-18s. Television programmes, magazines, comics, videos, films, recorded music and radio broadcasts targeted at children and adolescents are to be found in abundance. Advertising promotions directed at children can be found in all the media. Those who work within the media would appear to believe that their products can exert an influence. This belief is demonstrated in the continuing production of 'educational' programmes such as *Sesame Street* and in the recent appearance of psychological or educational consultants in the credits of cartoons such as *Thundercats* and comedies such as *The Cosby Show*. It is also shown in the 'nine o'clock watershed' adhered to by the BBC and commercial television channels as a guideline for the broadcasting of explicit programming (usually related to sex, violence or 'bad language'). The BBC also issues guidelines to production staff (BBC Television, 1987) on the possible effects of violence on children, urging caution regarding the use of excessively violent images in drama as well as documentary programmes.

People outside the media also appear to believe in this power to affect development. This belief is perhaps most clearly demonstrated with regard to the undesirable effects which the mass media are seen as exerting. Indeed, as Gunter (1986) notes with regard to television, there seems to be a tendency amongst mass communications researchers to look for negative effects. It is certainly not difficult to list the negative effects which are often associated with the media. The portrayal of violence, stereotypes and 'anti-social' behaviours, the encouragement of dangerous imitative behaviours, the spreading of obscene or blasphemous ideas or activities are all possible effects which have received heavy criticism. But positive roles for the media are also possible.

The Effects of the Media

Printed media

Reading is generally viewed as a positive activity for children. According to Mackey (1991), reading helps children to 'locate themselves in the world', with the narrative of literature illuminating a child's development as an individual in society. For Stones (1983), children's literature is important for sex-role socialisation, for the acquisition of gender identity. Other writers support children's magazines. McRobbie (1991) notes a new realism in what she sees as the best of the 1990s' crop of girls' magazines. Such publications, McRobbie suggests, have a 'focus on the self'. They credit teenage girls with more intelligence than magazines have previously and focus to a greater extent on job and career issues. The new realism also results in an acknowledgement by some magazines that many of their under 16-year-old readers will be sexually active and will have a greater ability to deal with subjects such as child abuse.

Comics, the most maligned of the printed forms, also have their supporters. Stan Lee, the Editor-in-Chief of Marvel Comics (publishers of 'Spiderman', 'The Incredible Hulk' and 'X-Men'), claims that comics are 'like the last bastion of defence against creeping illiteracy. A comic book is one of the few things that a youngster will read without being forced to, and getting kids to read anything is quite an achievement' (quoted in Connolly, 1991). Comics combine the narrative of the short story with the power of visual images, whether in full length super-hero adventures or in the single-page sagas of Dennis the Menace or Desperate Dan. This combination is a powerful one and has helped to maintain comics' popularity with children for many years. It is also an enduring one: comics remain popular with many readers well into adult life (Connolly, 1991).

Television and other broadcast media are criticised for their part in reducing the amount of printed media read by children. This criticism stems from the notion that TV is 'bad' and printed media are 'good'. What is often forgotten is the body of research which criticises these same printed media for their own supposedly detrimental effects on children's development, particularly through stereotyping, especially of gender and race. Stones (1983) identified numerous examples of sexism in publications for children, and emphasised her concern that such sexism creates a view of society where options are more limited by gender typing than in real life.

Sound effects

For children and teenagers, the medium of sound invariably means music – music listened to alone, as an 'isolator' via the personal stereo, as an accompaniment to shopping, work, exam revision or socialising, or as the focus of entertainment at live performances. It is popular music, in any of its constantly expanding subdivisions such as rap, heavy metal, house or soul, which is particularly important to the young, and it is popular music whose possible effects have generated concern.

With regard to its effects on development, the concerns raised relate not to the music itself but to the accompanying lyrics. The

Committee on Communications of the American Academy of Pediatrics (1989) showed particular concern about what it saw as the increasing explicitness of lyrics, especially those referring to sex and drugs and communicating 'potentially harmful messages'. The Committee proposed the idea that the public, especially parents, should be made aware of 'explicit lyrics', an idea that has been adopted in the United States and Britain by means of stickers on some record sleeves indicating the presence of such lyrics. Song lyrics, particularly when combined with new musical forms, have often aroused controversy and calls for their banning. The proposal of the Committee on Communications is only one recent example in a long line stretching back to the early days of rock'n'roll, and is highly unlikely to be the last.

The one-eyed monster

Only a brief search through the literature is needed to discover the real media 'villain'. Television has attracted many more times the attention from media researchers than all other forms combined: and in the majority of cases it is seen indeed as the 'one-eyed monster' (Gunter and McAleer, 1990). But what exactly does television (and its younger technological sibling the

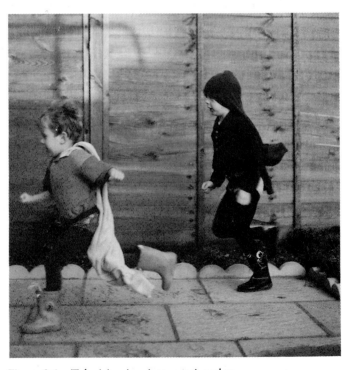

Figure 3.1   Television inspires creative play

video-recorder) do to children? The influences attributed to television include many already noted for other media. The difference appears to be that television, more than any other medium, is all-pervading in its presence. Television is there, in your home, available at the push of a button and assaulting your eyes and ears at once. It makes no 'complex demands on either mind or behaviour' (Postman, 1983). Ninety-eight per cent of British homes have a TV set, many possessing two or more (Gunter and McAleer, 1990). In the United States the average TV is switched on for over seven hours a day (Liebert and Sprafkin, 1988). It is possible to watch TV twenty-four hours a day, with at least four channels to choose from and an almost inexhaustible selection of video-recordings if the broadcast programmes do not appeal. We see and hear television simultaneously and, unlike books or comics, which parents can scan through before their children read them, you can never quite guarantee what's coming next.

Children are likely to be exposed to television output from the early days of their lives and, according to some research evidence, to be influenced by this output from an early age. Meltzoff (1988) found that children as young as 14 months old can imitate actions seen on television not only as they happen but also later on, even when a significant period elapses between the viewing of the action (in this case the manipulation of a specially designed toy) and the first opportunity to copy the action: a process termed 'deferred imitation'. What is significant in Meltzoff's work, apart from the idea that TV can influence even toddlers' behaviours, is that television's images are two-dimensional and yet they can be interpreted by young children to enable them to 'guide their own three-dimensional behaviour in the world'.

By 3 years of age children seem to be establishing definite viewing patterns and exercising preferences for what to watch. Liebert and Sprafkin (1988) suggest that by 4 years of age the average American child is watching television for 2.5 hours a day, with the amount of viewing peaking at four hours per day for the average 11-year-old. These figures are supported by the study by Huston *et al.* (1990) of two groups of children, aged 3 and 5 years respectively at the beginning of the two-year study. Average viewing per week was found to be about nineteen hours for the younger group and seventeen hours for the older: about 2.5–2.75 hours per day. This average does hide some substantially different examples of weekly viewing: in some instances children saw no TV in a week, on one occasion the researchers were given a recorded viewing time of 75.75 hours for a single week (or over ten hours per day).

Why do Children Watch Television?

Why do you watch television? To be entertained, educated, frightened, aroused? Because there's nothing better to do? Because you can't be bothered to get up and turn it off? Probably for all these reasons and more at one time or another. Children, too, have many reasons for watching TV or for choosing a particular programme. These reasons are well summarised by Gunter and McAleer (1990), who suggest:

- viewing as a habit or 'time-filler';
- viewing to learn (about social behaviour as well as about factual information);
- viewing for companionship (as a 'family activity' or to provide fantasy friends);
- TV as a babysitter;
- TV people as companions (forming 'para-social' relationships);
- TV as a source of conversation (a major reason for schoolchildren and adolescents, for whom it serves as a means of socialisation);
- viewing for escape;
- viewing as arousal;
- TV as mental or emotional stimulation to relieve boredom;
- viewing to improve bad moods, to 'feel better';
- TV as a source of reassurance and comfort.

Children are therefore active viewers, contrary to the tendency in much research to see them as passively receptive with viewing as an activity outside their lives (Gunter, 1986). Children choose to watch television to help themselves make sense of the world and to function more effectively within it. They also watch to cushion themselves from the less enjoyable elements of life: the boredom and the problems. TV also helps a child to identify with others: social interaction is supported by television viewing through its provision of common themes for discussion or common interests – television as friendly robot rather than one-eyed monster.

How do Children Watch TV?

As well as being active in deciding what to watch, children are active in how they watch. This active nature makes it particularly difficult to arrive at an accurate assessment of the length of time children watch TV. Huston *et al.* (1990) noted in their study of viewing patterns that a child's presence in a room while a TV is switched on does not truly reflect their attention to it. Fishbein (1987) found that pre-school children would turn away or be distracted more than 150 times during a single programme.

Active viewing depends on factors such as the programme's format, particularly the ease with which it can be followed and understood. This is itself mainly dependent on a child's age (Gunter and McAleer, 1990), with increasing knowledge being an important reason for age-related changes in viewing habits (Huston *et al.*, 1990). Huston's study identified other age-related aspects of viewing preference. Cartoons were most popular with 3–5-year-olds, with older children preferring 'general audience' comedies. The gender of the child also influences preferences, with children as young as 5 or 6 years old showing a greater liking for own-sex characters – although Gunter (1986) also notes that male characters receive more attention from children of both sexes than do female characters, while boys preferred more cartoon, informative 'adult audience' and action adventure shows than did girls.

What do children see?

Watching television day in and day out, year in and year out, the average 1990s' child is likely to have seen upwards of 15,000 hours of broadcasts and videotapes before leaving school. Quite apart from concerns about the sheer quantity of viewing, the major worries raised by academic and popular press alike centre on what children see when they watch.

The presentation of stereotypes

The use of stereotypes in television programmes is well documented. In a review of studies of programme content Gunter (1986) concludes that there is 'a persistent sexism in the portrayal of women and men on television'. He also notes that women on television are 'grossly outnumbered' by men and have a more limited range of roles. Bee (1989) identifies male TV characters as more active, aggressive and independent than females, with only the characteristics of deference and passivity being shown by women more often than men. She also draws our attention to the role played by many female characters: the 'handmaiden' to the more active and independent male (for example, in the traditional TV portrayals of doctor–nurse relationships).

Lewis and Volkmar (1990) also suggest that women TV characters are normally dominated by male characters. They also note that single women are likelier victims of aggression in TV drama than are married women, and that employed women are more likely to be portrayed as crooks than are those who are shown as housewives. They also identify racial stereotyping in TV drama, with non-whites being portrayed as subordinate to, smaller and less important than white characters and as criminals and victims.

TV Violence

The world of television is a violent world. In Liebert and Sprafkin's words, TV shows us that the world is 'a mean and scary place' (1988). TV violence is also tremendously varied in its scope. At one end of the spectrum cartoon characters regularly inflict extreme violence on one another with guns, bombs, blunt instruments, cars and all other possible sources to find that such violence serves to halt their adversaries only for an instant. Children's adventure series such as *The A-Team* or *The Incredible Hulk* use similar cartoon-like violence where victims emerge only slightly shaken from explosions, car wrecks or machine-gun attacks. More realistic dramas make regular use of violent acts and clearly depict them as causing pain, fear and injury to their recipients. The ultimate result of aggression, violent death, is to be found in often graphic detail on TV news and current affairs programmes.

Images of violence

Fifteen years ago Eysenck and Nias, while calling for further, better quality research, felt confident enough to write:

> The evidence is fairly unanimous that *aggressive acts new to the subject's repertoire of responses, as well as acts already well established, can be evoked by the viewing of violent scenes portrayed on film, TV, or in the theatre.*
>
> (1978: 252, their emphasis)

Ten years later Liebert and Sprafkin (1988) suggested that research 'continues to provide evidence of a causal relationship between violence viewing and aggression'. Other authorities

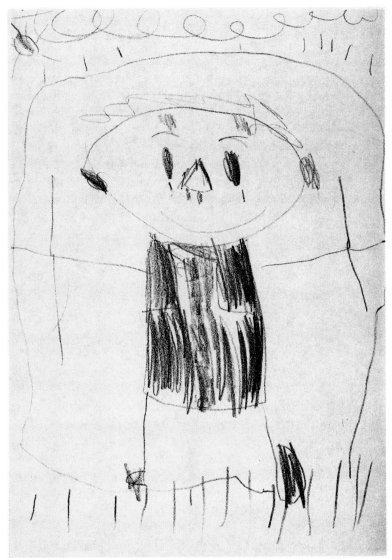

Figure 3.2 'A dead Cavalier waiting to be buried after being shot. He is smiling because he was told a very funny joke just before he died.' Drawn by Sam, aged 4½ years, some months after seeing a TV programme in which the character was featured. An example of the malignant influence of television, or simply of 'learning through viewing'?

have sounded a more cautious note about this supposed 'causal relationship', questioning the research methodologies used and the tendency, particularly in laboratory experiments, to study the viewing of violence in a falsely induced social isolation. So to what extent can we be confident about the influence of media violence on children?

In their review of twenty field experiments related to the effects of violence viewing on children from pre-school to adolescence, Gadow and Sprafkin (1989) conclude that laboratory experiments tend to provide evidence for the development of three types of aggression: object aggression, directed against inanimate things (especially dolls and other toys); symbolic aggression, involving aggressive play (for example, with toy guns); and verbal aggression, including swearing or threats. Genuine hurtful physical aggression as a result of media influence was not examined or supported by these studies (if for no other reason than that there are obvious ethical problems in developing research protocols which would seek to initiate such aggression). Gadow and Sprafkin's major criticism of laboratory experiments centres on a crucial element of the environments they create: laboratories have no 'natural deterrents' for aggressive behaviour.

The field studies revealed by Gadow and Sprafkin were found to offer little support for the idea that media violence provokes or promotes aggression in the viewer. The reviewers suggest that judgement be reserved for the present. A second review of research literature, by Heath *et al.* (1989), also recommends caution. While they suggest that a 'modest but genuine' causal link exists between media violence and actual violence, they also note that the precise relationship is too complex and has too many questions to be clearly understood. The possible effects of media violence are classified as 'behavioural' or 'attitudinal'; the strengths of each are found by Heath and her team to vary.

Behavioural effects help to create or develop aggressive or violent behaviours in children. Attitudinal effects include desensitisation, disinhibition towards aggression, increased fear and anxiety. Heath *et al.* identify a link between viewing violence and aggressive behaviour, and also comment that high exposure to televised violence can alter a child's perception of the world. This altered perception was identified as particularly apparent where direct experience by the child was unlikely, distorting the child's world-view and creating fear. They note, however, that no evidence was found that viewing TV violence makes children 'harder' or more callous.

One comment from Gadow and Sprafkin (1990) in a letter in support of their 1989 study is especially noteworthy. Their study of field experiments showed, they claim, that 'both aggressive- and nonaggressive-content media are likely to induce anti-social behaviour and that in a surprising number of studies the latter produced the higher level of aggression'. In other words, the simple act of watching television could alter a child's behaviour. As Gadow and Sprafkin state, 'television is "hot"' (1989).

Creating Change? Responding to the Effects of the Media

The mass media do seem to have the potential to affect the development of children in substantial ways. However, more discussion is needed before we can reach any effective conclusions regarding the precise nature and degree of these effects and the ways in which we as health professionals could or should respond to them. This section will go on to consider the possible effects and discuss the mediating influence of interactions between the different media and between the media and some important external factors.

Media effects on development: a summary

The media stand accused of exerting undesirable influences in four areas, outlined below. But for each area it is also possible to identify positive influences. This contrast results in some interesting comparisons.

First, the mass media occupy time which a child could use for more interactive, demanding and worthwhile activities. Too much time in front of the TV, or reading, or listening to music is harmful to the development of, for example, social or behavioural skills.

Fishbein (1987) suggests that, in fact, the media tend to cancel one another out in terms of time spent in consuming them. His work on children and television revealed that when children chose to watch TV the activities which suffered most as a result were radio-listening, movie-going and reading. Activities such as spending time with friends, sports, hobbies and personal interests were not affected.

Secondly, the mass media promote undesirable stereotypes and world-views which are unrepresentative of the 'real world' and which can lead to prejudiced attitudes and discriminatory approaches to others.

The literature contains many examples of media stereotypes and notes that race, gender and role are often portrayed in unrealistic ways. The media emphasis on violence and its need to depict exciting and novel acts as occurring far more frequently than would be the case in the real world tends to present a distorted view of the world and can influence children and young people in their views of it.

Nurses are frequently portrayed stereotypically in the media, with TV, cinema and the printed media offering children a series of unrepresentative images. Bridges (1990) identified four media images of nurses, all derogatory: the 'ministering angel', 'battleaxe matron', 'sex symbol' and 'doctor's handmaiden'. In addition, she noted, nurses are stereotypically white, female and single. It also seems clear that the vast majority of media nurses work in hospital, caring for the acutely physically ill patient. A child whose experience of nurses is gained from such media representations is likely to develop a similarly narrow and un-representative concept of nurses and nursing.

The mass media do focus on more optimistic elements of life, however, and can present much more positive representations of, for example, women or people from ethnic groups. Gunter (1986) notes that counter-stereotyping in the media may help to produce positive changes in the ways young people view the sexes. Fishbein (1987) suggests that TV viewing can have a pos-itive effect on cognitive growth in young children (although he also indicates that teenagers with a high level of TV viewing tend to have lower levels of academic achievement) and can positively influence social beliefs and behaviours. Stones (1983) emphasises the role non-sexist literature can have in helping children to achieve 'full intellectual and social development by freeing them from constricting ideas of what women and men can do'.

There is also more recent evidence to suggest that the media are indeed moving towards more positive portrayals. McRob-bie's observations about modern girls' magazines (1991) have already been discussed: she also identifies a growing tendency towards counter-stereotyping in popular children's programmes and soap operas such as *Grange Hill*, *Brookside* and *Neigh-bours*. In these programmes girls are strong-minded, independent and assertive, while boys are shown as having feel-ings as well as enjoying more traditionally masculine activities. McRobbie also suggests that girls are much more equal within relationships in the fictional media than was the case ten years ago.

Media representations of nurses are also changing, with pro-grammes such as BBC's *Casualty* offering much more realistic portrayals, including nurses who are male, black, married, and showing nurses as decision makers. One programme, ITV's *Children's Ward*, is targeted specifically at children and portrays many different representations of nurses. Such programmes may well do much to develop a better understanding of health care amongst young people.

Thirdly, the mass media aid consumerism through marketing strategies aimed specifically at the young. Children and teenagers are a major target for advertisers, particularly around Christmas. Lewis and Volkmar (1990) note that an average child in the United States will watch more than 20,000 TV commercials in a single year. The majority of commercials targeted at young viewers are for sweets and snack foods, with toys and games taking up much of the remaining time (Bernard-Bonnin *et al.*, 1988). Comics and magazines also include advertisements targeted at this market. More insidiously, children are exposed to advertisements for alcohol and tobacco products in shop windows and on billboards and hoardings. This exposure may help to promote the continued uptake of under-age drinking and cigarette smoking despite other attempts at the restriction of advertisements for such products.

Recent years have seen the development of a subtler form of commercialism. Consumer goods such as toys, models, games and clothes which relate to media characters are now big business. The promotion of these goods comes not through advertisements but through the programmes and magazines featuring the characters. Connolly (1991) states that television and cinema productions have an 'overriding influence' on sales. Such an influence is well demonstrated by the *Teenage Mutant Ninja Turtles* characters. Originally created as a comic, the cartoon series came to Britain in the late 1980s and was followed by dozens of commercial products. Their success was phenomenal but brief, lasting less than two years. By the end of 1992, while the Turtles still appear on British TV, the market has been taken over by others such as American wrestlers and the 1960s puppet adventure series *Thunderbirds*.

The effect of marketing is of particular concern in relation to young children. Lewis and Volkmar (1990) note that pre-school children have difficulty differentiating between advertisements and programmes on TV. As the boundary between advertisements and programmes blurs, with many children's characters seemingly created primarily to promote a product, such a differentiation may well become redundant.

If advertising in the media can have an effect on children's consumption of sweets, clothes and drinks, then it seems obvious that these same media can be used to influence children's behaviours with regard to, for example, diet or drug use. Certainly the possibilities for such a use are identified within the literature. Nutbeam *et al.* (1989) suggest that the mass media have a vital part to play in 'raising awareness about issues, providing role models and reinforcement for behavioural intentions', either in national strategies or in combination with localised health promotion programmes. The Committee on Communications of the American Academy of Pediatrics (1989) suggest that rock performers should be encouraged to act as positive role models and that the video and music industries should be encouraged to produce 'pro-social' videos.

Karpf (1988) cites evidence to show that American teenage girls reduced their use, or changed their brand, of tampons following publicity in US media about toxic shock syndrome. But she also notes a general failure of health education programmes in the media. As an example she cites the British anti-heroin campaign of 1985–86 which reportedly 'made the drug a challenge to some young people, ... the province of pale young anti-heroes'.

Fourthly, the mass media encourage young people to develop 'anti-social' behaviours. The media, particularly television, include a large amount of violence. Other elements are also criticised, such as swearing, blasphemy, or the portrayal of sexual acts (BBC Television, 1987). Research evidence suggests that the portrayal of violence in the media can lead to an increase in violent behaviour in children as well as to a change in children's attitudes to such things as the acceptability of violence as a means of achieving goals (Bee, 1989).

The research into the link between anti-social behaviour and the mass media does not present us with clear and unequivocal evidence. However, if there is a link between the media and anti-social behaviour, then can it be assumed that there is also a link between the media and pro-social behaviour? We have already discussed the possibilities of using the media to promote healthier behaviours in young people or to change their views of previously stereotyped roles, races or sexes. We have also considered the way in which literature and TV can help children to 'locate themselves in the world' (Mackey, 1991) or to solve problems in their everyday lives (Gunter and McAleer, 1990). So it seems likely that the media can influence the development of desirable as well as undesirable behaviours or attitudes (although exactly what should be defined as 'desirable' is often contentious). The exact nature and extent of this influence, as with most of the other influences we have considered, remains uncertain.

Interactions: the Reality of the Mass Media in Society

The mass media do not exist in isolation. What children see or hear is not solely the result of decisions made within the media. The reality of the relationship between the media and children is one of interactions.

Children can only see, hear or read what is made available by TV companies, publishers or the record industry. The decision to produce or broadcast something depends on many factors. One such factor is social acceptability: whether or not society will tolerate or allow something to be presented. Two or three decades ago children would have been exposed to frequent TV advertisements for cigarettes, while 'four-letter words' and nudity would have been virtually unknown in TV drama. Today all TV tobacco advertising is banned, but nudity and swearing are almost commonplace, even before the 'nine o'clock watershed'.

Commercialism also affects the media's plans for production. In most cases the media are seeking to make a profit and rely to a large extent on advertising revenue. Advertisers are unlikely to spend money to advertise during unpopular programmes or in low-circulation magazines, and so media executives need to cater to popular interests. Of course, this can also be seen as a way for children themselves to influence media output: if they do not like what the media make available, then they will not watch or buy it.

Planners' decisions regarding when to broadcast or publish also affect the availability of media product (Huston *et al.*, 1990), although in the case of TV programmes the use of video-recorders means that time of broadcast is no longer an effective means of preventing the viewing of a programme by young children (if indeed it ever was). So, too, do decisions about what to produce, which are based on reasons other than ones of social acceptability or commerce. The BBC, in its guidelines on TV violence (1987), urges caution in a number of areas, noting, for example, that 'It is never the case that only a targeted group of viewers is watching'. It advises its programme makers to avoid showing dangerous situations which children may easily imitate and cautions that 'what may appear self-evident to an adult will not necessarily have that same meaning for a child'.

Interactions within a child's social group are also likely to affect the child's use of the media. Children's socialisation may well include conversations about particular TV programmes. Similarly, a child's involvement in a peer group may be an influence on, or be influenced by, the individual child's choice of music or reading matter. Of particular importance is the role of the family structure and carers' activities in influencing use of the media. This role may vary from one where little or no attempt is made by parents to influence the child, to a very strict one where tight control is kept over access to television, books or the radio. Pinon *et al.* (1989), for example, in their study of the watching of *Sesame Street* by children in the United States found that family participation in school and work, the child's time in care facilities (crèches, nurseries) and the presence or absence of siblings were important influences. Parental encouragement led to high viewing of the programme.

Most important of all, perhaps, is the interaction between the individual child and the mass media. Although many authors, such as Anderson (1989), see television in particular as offering effects without exertion, the true picture appears to be radically different. As Rice and Woodsmall (1988) indicate, children are active processors of the media. They are participants in an interaction, rather than simply passive recipients of messages which they take on board unquestioningly (Gunter and McAleer, 1990).

It is important to note that the opportunity for interaction varies between the media. Self-exposure to TV, video and printed illustrations is likely to begin at a much earlier age than self-exposure to the written word (Heath *et al.*, 1989). This variation is seen by some authors as affecting the very nature of childhood itself. Meyrowitz (1985) criticises television for its lack of barriers to interaction, for its lack of 'complex access codes'. For him it is generally true to say that there are children's books and adults' books: the complexity of codes used, such as language and graphics, effectively excludes children from adult reading matter until they are able to understand and use these codes themselves. Television, he states, has no such codes, and there is, therefore, no such thing as adults' or children's television. Postman (1983) takes these concerns even further, believing that television erodes the difference between childhood and adulthood because of its 'undifferentiated accessibility'. The electronic media, claims Postman, find it impossible to withhold any secrets: 'Without secrets, of course, there can be no such thing as childhood'.

Responding to the Media: Strategies for the Family and the Health Professional

So how, if at all, should health professionals respond to the media in caring for children? Suggested responses in the literature range from involvement at a national level in policy making to the advising of parents regarding the exercising of control over a child's access to the media. In almost all cases the suggestions are applied to television.

Involvement at a national level is proposed by a number of authors. Lewis and Volkmar (1990) suggest that a national policy on TV violence may be of use in the United States. Bernard-Bonnin *et al.* (1988) conclude from their Canadian study that paediatricians should act politically to influence television output. The Committee on Communications of the American Academy of Pediatrics (1989) believe (somewhat naïvely, I feel) that what they see as the problem of explicit lyrics and images can be solved through 'Good taste and self-regulation by consumers, media, and the music industry', although they also suggest a national programme to inform the public of explicit content in music or videos. Proposals are put forward in the literature for local-level strategies to optimise the media's beneficial effects, or at least to minimise their undesirable ones. For health professionals, the first strategy is one which on the surface seems obvious but which rarely seems to be adopted by those who show most concern. Try to experience the same media that children experience: watch children's TV, read their comics and magazines, listen to the music which they listen to. Both Anderson (1989) and Bernard-Bonnin *et al.* (1988) support this strategy, which has the important benefit of being enjoyable and is likely to provide you with greater insight into why particular programmes, musical styles or magazines are important to a child. It will also help you to understand the mixture of media inputs experienced by individual children and hence to understand their life experiences better.

There are three other strategies which are worthy of consideration by health professionals with responsibility for children (for example, in residential care or as hospital in-patients) and for parents or carers in the child's home environment. First, monitor media use; understand the importance of the various media for a particular child. Get to know what media are used, to what extent and in what ways.

Secondly, 'co-consume'. Share TV viewing, read books or magazines, listen to music with the child (Bee, 1989; Bernard-Bonnin, 1988). Not only will you develop your understanding of the child's relationship with the media, but you will also let the child know this. Some children may well decide that anything an adult is interested in can't be that good and will move on. But many others will take your interest in what they watch or read as interest in them, to the benefit of your relationship with the child.

Thirdly, discuss what is presented in the media with the child (Bee, 1989; Lewis and Volkmar, 1990). Discussion allows each of you to indicate your own feelings about programmes, magazines or music. It enables you to indicate approval or disapproval, or to emphasise particular aspects of a story or lyric which you value or condemn. A discussion allows adult and child to defend personal views about, for example, the merits of a cartoon super-hero: even toddlers can present a vigorous argument in support of a favourite character or song. Use discussion to balance the bias of a programme or article, or to point out the unreality of a plot or action, or to identify how a particularly spectacular or fantastic or unpleasant act which may appear glamorous in media fiction would occur in real life. Discussion can help to place the media usefully within the context of a child's life, giving it a positive role as an influence on development.

A fourth strategy is proposed by many authors, including Bee (1989) and Bernard-Bonnin (1988): control of access to the media. There are problems with this strategy for two main reasons: its possibility and its value. Although control of access to the television, video-recorder or hi-fi may be possible in some homes, it may well serve only to drive a child to seek access elsewhere. Indeed, it may increase the desire to seek that access as the unavailability of a programme or film increases its desirability for the child. The value of controlling access is particularly questionable when it equates simply to prevention. Successful prevention denies the child an experience. Unsuccessful prevention, where the child gains access without the carer's knowledge, denies the carer the possibility of using the experience positively. If you feel strongly enough that a child should be prevented from watching, reading or listening to something, then whenever possible you should discuss your reasons. Once again, even young children can understand an argument which is appropriately put across, although they are not guaranteed to accept it.

If you are advising parents about using the mass media, remember to be realistic in your expectations. Anderson (1989) may advise against using TV as a babysitter, but for many parents it appears excellent in that role. Advising reduction in its use, rather than a complete stop, is more achievable. It is also worth remembering that the mass media are a part of the child's environment: completely preventing access to one of them may help to exclude a child from important aspects of everyday life. The resulting social isolation may be less desirable than the apparent over-exposure to the media which you have sought to prevent.

Future Developments?

The discussion in this chapter has focused on the role of the media in certain aspects of child development, highlighting those which may be of particular importance to those of us who nurse children. The media, especially TV, affect the lives of almost all children in contemporary Western society and are likely to do so for the foreseeable future. However, like many other aspects of children's lives, the media are changing, and these changes raise new issues regarding development. The growth of TV channels and video-recordings means that children now have a much greater range of things to watch, reducing the likelihood of one programme or film being popular across a large proportion of children.

Perhaps most importantly, modern technology has produced something which may significantly threaten the importance of the media in children's lives. Computer games are now a major leisure pursuit among school-age children and sell in their millions in Britain, the United States and elsewhere, while many children are more deeply involved in computer operating and

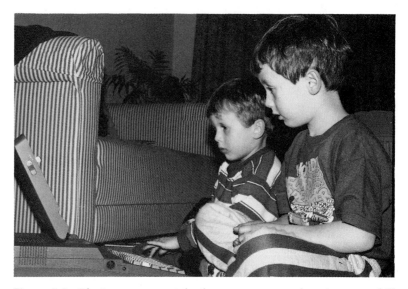

Figure 3.3 Playing games on the laptop computer: learning new skills through new technology

programming. Computers offer children a vast range of possibilities in terms of enjoyment, education and future careers. Their effects on development are as yet virtually unknown, with current research offering an inadequate grasp of the possibilities (Crook, 1992).

For child health care the possibilities of computer technology appear almost infinite. Do we expect a future full of isolated adolescents with poor social skills, hunched over computer keyboards for the bulk of their leisure hours, or will we see the opening up for the young of new methods of communication and social interaction? In either case, children's nurses must be sure to understand what this new technology means for child development in health.

References

Anderson, J. J. T. (1989) 'Developing children', in R. L. R. Foster, M. M. Hunsberger and J. J. T. Anderson (eds) *Family-centred Nursing Care of Children*, Philadelphia: W. B. Saunders.

BBC Television (1987) *Violence on Television: Guidelines for Production Staff*, London: BBC Publications.

Bee, H. (1989) *The Developing Child*, 5th edn, New York: Harper and Row.

Bernard-Bonnin, A-C., Gilbert, S., Rousseau, E., Masson, P. and Maheux, B. (1988) 'Television and the 3- to 10-year-old child', *Pediatrics*, 1: 48.

Bridges, J. M. (1990) 'Literature review on the images of the nurse and nursing in the media', *Journal of Advanced Nursing*, 15: 850.

Committee on Communications of the American Academy of Pediatrics (1989) 'Impact of rock lyrics and music videos on children and youth', *Pediatrics*, 2: 314.

Connolly, J. (1991) 'Soul-kiss of the Spiderman', *The Times Saturday Review*, 26 October, p. 6.

Crook, C. (1992) 'Cultural artefacts in social development: the case of computers', in H. McGurk (ed.) *Childhood Social Development: Contemporary Perspectives*, Hove: Lawrence Erlbaum Associates.

Eysenck, H. J. and Nias, D. K. B. (1978) *Sex, Violence and the Media*, London: Maurice Temple Smith Ltd.

Fishbein, H. (1987) 'Socialization and television', in O. Boyd-Barrett and P. Braham (eds) *Media, Knowledge and Power*, London: Croom Helm.

Gadow, K. D. and Sprafkin, J. (1989) 'Field experiments of television violence with children: evidence for an environmental hazard?' *Pediatrics*, 83(3): 399.

Gadow, K. D. and Sprafkin, J. (1990) 'Television violence' (letter), *Archives of General Psychiatry*, 47: 595.

Gunter, B. (1986) *Television and Sex Role Stereotyping*, London: John Libbey and Co. Ltd.

Gunter, B. and McAleer, J. L. (1990) *Children and Television: the One-eyed Monster?* London: Routledge.

Heath, L., Bresolin, L. B. and Rinaldi, R. C. (1989) 'Effects of media violence on children: a review of the literature', *Archives of General Psychiatry*, 46: 376.

Huston, A. C., Wright, J. C., Rice, M. L., Kerman, D. and St Peters, M.

(1990) 'Development of television viewing patterns in early childhood: a longitudinal investigation', *Developmental Psychology*, 26(3): 409.

Karpf, A. (1988) *Doctoring the Media: the Reporting of Health and Medicine*, London: Routledge.

Lewis, M. and Volkmar, F. (1990) *Clinical Aspects of Child and Adolescent Development*, 3rd edn, Philadelphia: Lea and Febiger.

Liebert, R. M. and Sprafkin, J. (1988) *The Early Window: Effects of Television on Children and Youth*, 3rd edn, New York: Pergamon Press.

Mackey, M. (1991) 'Ramona the chronotype: the young reader and social theories of narrative', *Children's Literature in Education*, 22(2): 97.

McRobbie, A. (1991) *Feminism and Youth Culture: From 'Jackie' to 'Just Seventeen'*, Basingstoke: Macmillan.

Meltzoff, A. N. (1988) 'Imitation of televised models by infants', *Child Development*, 59: 1221.

Meyrowitz, J. (1985) *No Sense of Place: the Impact of Electronic Media on Social Behaviour*, New York: Oxford University Press.

Nutbeam, D., Aar, L. and Catford, J. (1989) 'Understanding children's health behaviour: the implications for health promotion for young people', *Social Science and Medicine*, 29(3): 317.

Pinon, M. F., Huston, A. C. and Wright, J. C. (1989) 'Family ecology and child characteristics that predict young children's educational television viewing', *Child Development*, 60: 846.

Postman, N. (1983) *The Disappearance of Childhood*, London: W. H. Allen.

Rice, M. L. and Woodsmall, L. (1988) 'Lessons from television: children's word learning when viewing', *Child Development*, 59: 420.

Stones, R. (1983) *'Pour Out the Cocoa: Janet': Sexism in Children's Books*, York: Longman for Schools Council.

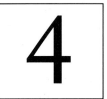

CHILDREN AND POWER

Terry Phillips
University of East Anglia

Children as Small Adults: the Historical Context

Childhood is a relatively modern invention. The question of what rights and responsibilities an adult has with respect to children, and vice versa, is still being worked out in the late twentieth century. Until the Children Act (1989) reversed the trend, changes in perceptions of childhood since the eighteenth century had systematically reduced the power children have over their own minds and bodies, and created an inversely proportionate increase in adult power. As society has moved from a position where the child was indistinguishable from the adult in terms of domestic and labour roles, through a position where the child was romanticised as 'better than' the adult, to the postmodern position where there is no unified view of what a child is, adults have continued to increase their power to determine children's lives for them. Improvements in physical care have been marked by a decline in children's active, subjective involvement in control over the processes which most directly affect their physical and intellectual health.

Until the late seventeenth century there was no differentiation between children and adults in daily life; children were treated as small adults in every respect. In the home they shared all the spaces with adults, including the sleeping areas; there were no rooms designated especially for children's activities, and no separate children's bedrooms. They wore exactly the same clothes as the adults, although in scaled-down versions, and did the same work in the fields or in the home. They would rise early with the adults and go to bed when they did. Life was governed for children and adults alike by the seasons and by religious or pagan festivals. Children were full members of the neighbourhood community of people living in the 'home' village, a community which was in effect an extended family with whom the child worked, played and lived. Children were less strong than adults, but, after allowances were made for that fact, they were accepted as equal participants in all aspects of life.

The integration of children's and adult's lives in seventeenth-century England had both positive and negative consequences for the children. On the one hand, they shared the celebrations and the corporate sense of achievement which occurred when the liturgy of church or nature marked the end of winter, or a safe harvest, or renewal of life at Easter. At seasonal festivities adults and children indulged together in the playfulness and innuendo which characterised such occasions. At other times they played the same games of hide-and-seek, blind man's buff, hopscotch and hoop whipping. None of these things had yet been marked out either as 'childish', and therefore to be put away as maturity approached, or 'too adult', and so to be kept from children for fear of corrupting them. On the other hand, children were subject to the same coarseness of behaviour, privy to the same sexual play, and subject to the same punishments as adults themselves. As they were not seen as anything other than small adults there was no attempt to shelter them from the debauchery that often accompanied street carnivals and fairs, or to protect them from excessive demands on their physical labour. The child who worked alongside adults pitching hay would be expected to work equal hours but to carry slightly lighter loads. The child who was apprenticed would be expected to do many of the more arduous tasks as a way of learning their craft. The child who was in domestic service would cook, sew and clean for as long as any of the adults. And irrespective of whether they were pursuing an agricultural, domestic or craft labour, the young would be expected to stop work when everyone else did, to eat the same meals, drink the same wine and share the same conversations. Before the eighteenth century the community's expectations of children and adults were identical.

In the late twentieth century we *permit* our children to join in adult activities from time to time, and give them, as it were, licence to behave differently on special occasions such as weddings and parties. In the period before the concept of childhood

had meaning it made no sense to *allow* children such privileges;
they had them by right. Children were adults in the sight of the
law from a very early age. Adult permission did not actually
have to be sought, because children were seen by law as responsible for their own actions. Under Tudor law, for instance, any
child aged 7 or over who was convicted of stealing could be
hanged. We know from contemporary written accounts that
children could and frequently did watch hangings, and accepted
them not only as a normal part of street life but also as the just
fate of *anyone* convicted of serious crime. In the late seventeenth
century, as numerous parish records show, children of a family
caught contravening the law would be publicly whipped along
with their parents. A child as young as 6 could and frequently
did become an apprentice in a household other than the
parents', but the law required that they should do so before
reaching 12. A boy could rise to the rank of lieutenant in the
army by the age of 14, and be responsible for the lives of others.
Society was not divided on the basis of chronological age but
according to able-bodiedness and economic viability.

To summarise, then, children's power or lack of it *vis-à-vis*
adults was not a conceivable issue before the eighteenth century.
The only members of a community who were segregated from
power were very young infants, the physically weak and the
incapacitated elderly, who, through inability to control their
own bodies, were forced to be dependent on others. Any fit
child who lived beyond infancy was assumed to be morally
responsible and capable of being economically productive and
was accorded the same social status as an adult. With this came
the power to control or be controlled, and of particular interest
from the point of view of the caring professions, to decide without reference to any adult what they did with and to their
bodies.

Dependent Infants and the Need for State Care

It is time to add a note of qualification. The picture presented so
far has suggested a cohesiveness to society's lack of distinction
between adults and children before the eighteenth century. Like
every other discourse, however, the sixteenth and seventeenth
century discourse about childhood was actually a lived debate
between competing ideologies. As individuals from different
communities met in the course of their daily lives, they brought
to their interactions a variety of perspectives on what constituted natural justice, and within that, a range of views about the

treatment of children. True, there was a dominant perspective, reiterated by the acts of work, survival and celebration as lived by the majority of people, but there were also sufficient alternative perspectives to maintain a constant challenge to the mainstream one. Although most people saw a world undifferentiated by age, and the greatest number of communities lived as if children were scaled-down adults, there was a significant minority who saw the young as different because of their physical vulnerability and consequent need for protection. This group was itself by no means a homogeneous one, but it did include several rich and powerful middle-class and aristocratic philanthropists, who had the economic and social power to act in ways that disturbed the dominant discourse. An alternative view of children was, then, already in place during the sixteenth and seventeenth centuries.

When a concept of children as dependents emerged it was one which secured popular support in several quarters. Although it did not immediately develop into an orthodoxy strong enough to affect adult–child interactions on a grand scale, but did challenge the dominant discourse. The idea of childhood was initiated by direct intervention rather than long-term persuasive argument, and happened to some extent within the framework of the dominant discourse. For it came about as a necessary part of finding a solution to a moral and economic dilemma that was actually created by the dominant discourse. Within a world view that treated adults and children alike, it became necessary to decide what should happen to those members of society who were so small and vulnerable that they could not be treated 'normally'; it became essential, in fact, to decide where children under 3 fitted into the picture. Before the eighteenth century, childhood equalled infancy, and a concern for the welfare of infants was what motivated the first distinction between adults' and children's rights and responsibilities.

The Invention of 'Childhood' and the Introduction of Education and Control

In the context of a society which in 1662 provided for its economically non-viable (amongst whom were many children) through Poor Laws that eventually led to the notorious conditions of the workhouse, the most notable move forward in the discourse about childhood happened with the setting up of Christ's Hospital in 1552, a charitable hospital intended to care for young orphans and offer them an education. With a generous one-to-sixteen carer–child ratio, Christ's Hospital cared for the orphans magnificently by providing them with comfortable accommodation, feather beds and plenty of food. By taking additional responsibility for education, however, the trustees extended the period of dependency beyond infancy for the first time. As an innovation is made in one discourse, a new orthodoxy may be caused in a parallel one. By recognising the need to provide care for the young, the founders of Christ's Hospital established childhood (for some at least) as that period of life during which adults have responsibility for children's welfare. By introducing schooling at the same time they also unwittingly made childhood a period of extended dependence and relative powerlessness for the children. As they received an education (which included learning to read and write in English, Latin and Greek, to do mathematics, and to develop skills in readiness for apprenticeships), children were taught to subject themselves to the will of adults in a way unknown to their peers growing up elsewhere in the community on equal terms with adults. The 'new' child was motivated extrinsically by adult entreaties to prepare for the future, rather than intrinsically by the task in hand, and they became a recipient of knowledge and skill rather than a participant in the use of them. The arrival of the first care-provision for children to be offered outside the extended family of the community brought into being a system of organised education and training which required control, and dramatically altered the power relationship between adults and children. John Evelyn wrote in 1687 after a visit to the Hospital: 'I saw them at supper, visited their dormitories, and much admired the order, economy, and excellent government of this most charitable seminary'. His comments emphasises the new relationship between those who order the child's world to protect them, and the children who are the recipients of the protection.

Increasing Asymmetry in the Adult–Child Power Relationship _____

The counter-discourse of childhood as 'difference from adulthood' described above continued to gain ground throughout the eighteenth century, and was moving towards the dominant position by the nineteenth. It never completely replaced the Enlightenment discourse of children as scaled-down adults; indeed, this exists today and can be recognised most readily in advertising that encourages children to see themselves as young adults, but it did alter the balance between that view and the view of children as people with different needs and rights from adults. The new balance marked a shift from adult–child equality to an asymmetry in adult–child power. This shift of balance is exemplified in such official actions as those of the judges who, from 1717 onwards, arranged to have hundreds of young child beggars deported to start a new life in Virginia, North America. By taking that action the judges not only demonstrated their humaneness but also marked out the young beggar as potentially different from adult beggars, as more able to benefit from a new start. The shift is also indicated by the increasing pressure on the London-based Thomas Coram Foundling Hospital between the time it was set up in 1740 and the latter part of the century. This Hospital drew on the wealth of private and parliamentary benefactors to care for large numbers of abandoned children. Like Christ's Hospital earlier, it introduced education alongside caring, and as its patrons included Handel, Reynolds and Hogarth, it was able to introduce its wards (the children in its care) to musical and artistic education as they grew older. Once again, however, in the process of providing care, the officers of the Hospital found it necessary to assume power over the children, ordering their lives for them in a way which would have been deemed inappropriate in earlier times. As the Hospital's statute stated: 'from that time [when the child is three and has returned from being cared for by a nurse in the country] until they are six years old [they should] be taught to read, learn the catechism, and at proper times exercise in the open air'.

The relationship between the provision of care and the adult assumption of control over children is encapsulated in the phrase 'at proper times', which suggests the introduction of a regime to improve health through outdoor activity that would once have happened in the course of working the land and living on the street. The power of adults to intervene in the health care of children who would previously have been thought free to care for (or neglect) themselves is further demonstrated by the fact that the carers at the Foundling Hospital could vaccinate the children for smallpox at the age of 3. There is no question that vaccination was a valuable instrument for controlling potentially lethal infectious diseases, which many observers might argue was in the interest of the child as well as of the rest of society, but it is interesting to note the connection between this adult intervention in children's health and the redistribution of power in the adult–child relationship. With an increase in adult power to order children's time (for learning) and control children's bodies (to ensure quality health care), the distribution of power between adults and children shifted dramatically in the eighteenth century.

The separation of children and adults continued throughout the nineteenth and twentieth centuries as the locus of productivity moved from the land to the town, and from the home to specialised places of work. As factories developed and working-class men with specialised skills went to work in them, leaving women behind to work in the home, the children who stayed with their mothers became isolated from men and the world of factory work. The gulf which developed between working-class children of both sexes and the males in their families was considerable. The distance between middle-class children and *both* their parents was even greater. Middle-class men spent their days in business and commercial ventures, and their wives occupied theirs in ways which kept them apart from the children. In both cases (the working class and the middle class), adults compensated for the loss of their children by building sentimental pictures of the beauty of childhood as a Golden Age. In the middle-class nursery (a space dedicated like a monument to childhood) children were presented with structured learning materials through which they could play and learn at the same time. For the working class there were parks which offered structured play areas. To protect the Golden Age image of childhood the nursery and the parks were regulated and supervised, and unauthorised play was discouraged. As with all surveillance, however, it was impossible to police every open space and every moment of the child's play. Children demonstrated their power to resist adult control by playing on the street in dangerous but exciting environments, and by choosing their own gangs of playfellows. According to Firestone, play was co-opted as a means of repression (Firestone, 1971); but it was never successfully incorporated because by this time children's separation from adults was complete and they had developed the will to do different things even if it meant fighting for the opportunity.

The Concern for Child Welfare and Education, and the Development of Adult 'Moral Power'

It is already apparent that a study of the development of adult–child power relationships and their effect on child care must consider not only the events which helped to construct that relationship – its history – but must also encompass the ideas and debates which informed (or perhaps reflected) those events.

Because it is also clear that the development of welfare provision for children involved the parallel promotion of physical and mental health (although the earlier philosophers might have called the latter moral health), it now seems appropriate to look briefly at the views of some of the major philosophical movements on childhood.

Typical of the concept of childhood which emerged during the eighteenth century and persisted long afterwards was the one embodied in the 1767 publication of the first book published exclusively for (middle-class) children. John Newberry's *Little Pretty Pocket Book*, addressed to Little Master Tommy and Pretty Miss Polly, combined education and entertainment. Newberry, in the guise of Jack the Giant Killer, wrote to each of them separately extolling their good (that is, non-adult) behaviour:

> She [the nurse] says you are very honest and good humoured; that you don't swear, tell lies, nor say indecent words, and are always thankful when any body gives you good advice, that you never quarrel, nor do wicked things, as some other boys [girls] do.

Newberry's book presents a strange mixture of what might be considered childish and what could be seen as child-as-miniature adult. He offers amusing playthings, such as a two-tone ball and a pincushion with black and red pins to record good and bad behaviour, together with alphabet rhymes, fables and proverbs. He also offers children the prospect of perpetual surveillance:

> So live with men as if God's eye
> Did into every action pry,

and of punishment for misdemeanour:

> if ever the pins be all found on the black side of the ball, then I'll send a rod, and you shall be whipped as often as they are found there.

But by presenting his message in a form that was intended for the instruction and amusement of children, he contributed centrally to the reification of childhood. According to your perspective, the view of childhood which the *Little Pretty Pocket Book* represented either liberated children by acknowledging that emotionally and cognitively they experience the world differently from adults, or began the journey which condemned them for over 100 years to a mixture of sentimentality and brutality in the Victorian household, and which is present to some extent today.

Newberry's ideas about childhood derived a great deal from those of the philosopher and physician John Locke. Locke saw children as rational beings able to be convinced through reasoned argument, and although he saw reason as occasionally needing a back-up in the form of a beating (so that the child might learn and never need another!), he favoured entertainment and persuasion as methods for converting the ignorant child to wisdom.

> Without a sense of the shame or guilt of his [sic] action, the child will only be hardened in rebellion by physical punishment. Shame (and praise) help the child to internalise the parent's judgement. It impresses upon the child that the parent is not only more powerful, but right.
>
> (Locke, 1693)

Locke's educational philosophy, which was in fact a statement about the need for adults to base their authority over children on moral strength rather than physical coercion, asserted adult power and children's lack of it. The rational view was a humane one, but it constructed adults as supreme 'knowers' and children as subservient 'learners', and it presented coercion by means of moral blackmail as acceptable. For the man who wrote in his medical capacity in favour of loose swaddling, and against strict toilet training, there was still a case to be made for the restriction of a child's mental growth through guilt which would teach the child that the adult was right.

Demonstrating once again that there are always competing discourses within any culture, at about the same time as Locke's ideas were current, the very different perspective on childhood presented by Rousseau aroused the interest of philosophers across Europe. In 1762 Rousseau published *Emile* which depicted the child as a noble savage, an innocent who would be shaped not by adult intervention but by the forces of nature. According to Rousseau, the child's innocence would allow them to prosper and develop if unrestrained by the artificial frameworks of an increasingly corrupt society. Education and care of the child were to be carried out covertly so as not to inhibit the effect of nature, the natural teacher and healer. But there is no subjection so complete as that which appears to offer liberty without actually doing so. And Rousseau's concept of childhood, while differing in many ways from earlier ones which saw the child as sinful and in need of physical, moral and intellectual care to deliver it from the corruption of the world, nevertheless failed to reinstate the equality of power which had existed between children and adults before the century in which he and Locke were propagating their views.

The Exercise of Adult Power in Modern Child-care Nursing: Ways of Handing Power Back to the Child

This account of the historical and philosophical construction of childhood and of the power differential between adults and children helps us to realise that childhood 'is in large measure a social construction, the child is a modulated and modulating component in a shifting network of influences' (Berger and Luckmann, 1966), and that 'the child is essentially and eternally a cultural invention, and that the variety of the child's definition is not the removable error of an incomplete science' (Kessen, 1991). It alerts us to the necessity 'to disentangle the natural from the cultural' (Woodhead *et al.*, 1991), and reminds us that we must take care in resorting to a position which invokes a child's 'best interests' or refers to their 'needs' as we as late twentieth-century adults perceive them. Both the child's alleged best interests and their alleged needs are social constructions influenced by the fashionable requirements of the age.

Expectations influence possibilities. Just as some teachers in the past have perceived control over children to be essential if their learning is to be promoted in the least teacher-taxing way, so today's children's nurse may prefer the child who receives treatment without complaint and does what they are told because such a child makes it easier for the nurse to complete an often impossibly busy schedule. It takes less time to tell a child what to do than it does to consult them, and it is certainly easier for an adult to impose a course of action on a child than on another adult. This sort of action can have considerable and unfortunate consequences, however, for an adult who expects to invade a child's personal space and take control of their body without consultation with them will be inclined to reduce the child's autonomy further by discounting their view as one that needs to be taken into account. A vicious circle will be established, and the child will come to expect not to be responsible for their body whilst in a health-care context. By having a prior expectation that the child will not be able to do certain things and so intervening to do those things for them, the adult will 'construct' the child as incompetent. This raises a serious question about the nature of the adult–child health-care relationship, and the potential dangers of that relationship. In the words of Gideonse (1982):

> 'is it better to do for others if you can do better than they, or better to let them do for themselves even if the end result for the doer is not as complete, fulfilling, or "accurate"?'

Children have unexpected competence and resourcefulness if allowed the space to exercise it. This is an excellent reason for giving them that space. Another very compelling reason is that, if we begin to take it for granted that because the people we are dealing with are children we can call upon the power of our more extensive knowledge and the power of our greater experience to run their lives for them during their time in the caring environment, there is a danger that we will come to see ourselves as having the right to intervene and the child as having to claim the right to exercise control over its own mental and physical well-being if it wants it. To avoid this we must accept the view of Bartholome, writing in a US Department of Health and Welfare publication, that

> 'rights are not claims, they are entitlements, . . . they do not depend on the bearer possessing any relevant power or capacity. To have rights or entitlements it is only necessary for an individual to be a member of the group of rights-holding persons' (Bartholome, 1977)

and then go beyond that to agree with Hauerwas in the same publication that children's rights are a negative notion, placing all the responsibility on the child. With Hauerwas (1977) it is necessary to say that only by emphasising the *duty* of adults in caring situations where, by virtue of being adults they have an asymmetrical power, is it possible for nurses who care for children to avoid abusing their power.

References

Aries, P. (1962) *Centuries of Childhood: a Social History of Family Life*, Harmondsworth: Penguin.

Bartholome, W. G. (1977) 'Proxy consent in the medical context: the infant as person', in Appendix to *Research Involving Children*, (Document No. 77–0005), US Government Printing Office.

Berger, P. and Luckmann, T. (1966) *The Social Construction of Reality: a Treatise in the Sociology of Knowledge*, New York: Doubleday.

Borman, K. M. (ed.) (1982) *The Social Life of Children in a Changing Society*, Hillside, NJ: Lawrence Erlbaum Associates.

Firestone, S. (1971) *The Dialectic of Sex*, London: Jonathan Cape; reprinted in M. Hoyles (ed.) *Changing Childhood* (1979), London: Writers' and Readers' Co-operative.

Gideonse, H. D. (1982) 'The political uses of childhood', in K. M. Borman (ed.) *The Social Life of Children in a Changing Society*, Hillside, NJ: Lawrence Erlbaum Associates.

Hauerwas, S. (1977) 'Rights, duties, and experimentation on children: a critical response to Worsfold and Bartholome', in Appendix to *Research Involving Children* (Document No. 77–0005), US Government Printing Office.

Kessen, W. (1991) 'The American child and other cultural inventions', in M. Woodhead, P. Light and R. Carr (eds) *Growing Up in a Changing Society*, London: Routledge (in association with the Open University).

Locke, J. (1693) *Some Thoughts Concerning Childhood*, London.

Newberry, J. (1966) *A Little Pretty Pocket Book (Facsimile)*, London: Oxford University Press.

Woodhead, M., Light, P. and Carr, R. (eds) (1991) *Growing Up in a Changing Society*, London: Routledge (in association with the Open University).

PART 2

CONTEMPORARY CARE ISSUES

5 RESEARCH AND CHILD CARE

Jayne Taylor
Suffolk College

Health-care professionals working with children share one ultimate aim, which is simply that children and their families should receive the highest quality care. If that is not our ultimate aim, we are not only failing the consumers of the services we offer but we are also failing ourselves and our profession. Wanting children to have the best is not, however, a new phenomenon, and we must presume that our good intentions were shared with those professionals involved in the child health services, twenty, fifty and even 100 years ago, or more. And yet, research has shown us that many of the practices engaged in by our predecessors were at best of little use and, at worst, detrimental to the physical, psychological and social well-being of children.

It is always interesting to note the disbelief on student nurses' faces when they listen to how we used to 'care' for children. The shock of realising, for example, that children with tuberculosis and scarlet fever would be isolated from their families, often many miles from home, for weeks on end, makes us appreciate that children do not suffer similar fates in the 1990s. We must realise, however, that those health-care workers were doing what they considered to be 'the best' for those children and did not remove them from their homes and separate them from their families with the wish of making them suffer. High-quality care was their aim, just as it is ours. What we must do is to reflect on our practice every day of our working lives, and ask ourselves if any of our existing practices are useless or even harmful, or if indeed student nurses in fifty years' time will experience shock when they hear about our work.

This chapter examines research in child care and carries an overt message to anyone currently working with children or who wishes to do so in the future. The message is that if we do not look critically at our practice, if we do not use research in our work and if we do not seek out the best ways of delivering care to children, then inevitably we will have to face criticism in the future. We must, as professionals, be committed to developing the knowledge base which underpins practice and have the skills and desire to evaluate, discriminate and intelligently use that knowledge.

The Evolution of Practice

Looking through some rather ancient child nursing books can give us great insight into how research has shaped professional practice. For example, Myers (1910), in a book called *The Care of Children*, wrote about the treatment of the child with tonsillitis: 'gargles are of slight use, but painting with glycerine and tannin is more efficacious. The bowels must be kept open'. The obsession between bowels and tonsils persisted for many years, and Evelyn Pearce in her 1938 *Short Encyclopaedia for Nurses* commenced her section on the care of the patient with tonsillitis by writing: 'Rest in bed is essential, an aperient being given at the beginning of the illness, and the bowels kept active'. Without doubt, advances in medical and pathophysiological knowledge in many ways shaped the direction of nursing, and saved many children from frequent doses of castor oil and 'confection of sulphur'! Progress was, however, painfully slow and attitudes reluctant to change, particularly, it seems, when it came to the authority of the nurse over her small patients. An extract from a book by Lovely (1951), entitled *The Nursing of Sick Children*, illustrates this point. In a discussion about food refusal she writes: 'If food is refused, the less fuss made about it the better, and if water is withheld for a few days the child will usually take sufficient sweetened milk to keep him from harm' (p. 61).

There is a notable lack of reference to parents, although Lovely (1951), in what must have been a fairly innovative chapter at the time, entitled 'The psychological aspect of a children's ward', recommends that parents of older children may come and 'read to him for a short time each day'. Sadly, it was not research by nurses that led to change in parental access but psychologists such as Robertson and Robertson (in Robertson and Robertson, 1989) and Bowlby (1953) who examined the psychological effects of hospital on children and proclaimed that restricted visiting was a mistake and that parents, particularly mothers, should be encouraged to visit frequently and participate in the care of their children. Bowlby, in a later edition of his book *Child Care and the Growth of Love* (1965), also cited the innovative work of the hospitals in Newcastle upon Tyne and in New Zealand, where mothers were admitted with their young children. By this time the Platt Report (1959) had been published, which recommended that all new hospitals should be designed with facilities for parents, so that they might remain with their sick children. Unfortunately, later work by Poster (1983) and Rodin (1983) showed that, whilst many hospitals did have rooming-in and liberal visiting policies, the practice of what was actually happening did not reflect those policies. Parents were often unaware of the existence of facilities and, even if they knew such facilities were available, were ignorant of the importance of staying with their children. Part of the blame for this was placed with nurses, according to a Consumers' Association report (1985), which found that, whilst many children's wards advocated open visiting in theory, the practice was that parents were often made to feel unwelcome by staff. It is hoped that this situation has improved over the last few years, but we must ensure in future that it does not take thirty years to act on the findings of research.

Another major area of concern relating to children in hospital is the organisation of nursing staff. We still frequently hear from students that the nursing process, team and primary nursing systems are not functioning as efficiently as they should in some areas and that staff shortages sometimes result in task allocation rearing its head again, especially on late shifts and night duty. This is hardly ever meant as a criticism of busy nursing staff but of the organisation and managerial systems that proliferate within the health service today. Financial cut-backs inevitably mean staff cut-backs, and the reality on many wards is that the skill mix of staff dictates the organisation of staff rather than the needs of the children. The advancement of technology often means that the qualified nurses have to spend most of their time giving medications, caring for the intravenous infusions, checking ventilators and sorting out documentation, which leaves the remaining workforce (often sparse and relatively unqualified) engaged in undertaking a series of tasks. The effects on the children are obvious. They end up being cared for by a large number of different nurses and find it difficult to build relationships with anyone. And yet, even Bowlby (1965) wrote of the importance of individualised care, as did Cleary in 1977 and Weller in 1980. It appears that we are still not utilising research, even when we know that by not doing so we are failing the children in our care.

Utilisation of Research

We have already discussed some of the research from the fields of medicine, pathophysiology and psychology that have had an effect on our knowledge of nursing children in hospital. It is evident that as a profession, nursing reacts more readily to changes suggested as a result of medical research than it does to those made by psychologists. The reason for this willingness to change for doctors is not hard to guess at; the overt and covert power of doctors over nurses is still evident in (dare we say) most hospital wards today. Yet strangely, much of the nursing research which began to proliferate in the early 1970s has focused on the psychological needs of children in hospital and has frequently drawn on the theories of psychologists such as Bowlby. For example, Hawthorn's (1975) *Nurse, I Want My Mummy!*, Rodin's (1983) *Will This Hurt?*, Harris's (1979) *Children, Their Parents and Hospital*, and Brown's (1989) *Individualised Care* all focused on the necessity for nurses to consider the emotional needs of children. The questions we need to address are why nurses fail to use research findings, especially those emanating from members of their own profession or from psychologists, and why, according to Lynn (1989), less than 6 per cent of nursing knowledge is derived from scientific or systematically acquired knowledge. Hunt (1981) explains that the reluctance to utilise research has arisen because research is not known about, is not understood, believed, allowed or perceived to be relevant. Breu and Dracup (1976) believe that reluctance occurs because it involves change, and they suggest that resistance to change is a 'normal human response'. Breu and Dracup's suggestions do perhaps have even more relevance in the health service of the 1990s where there is almost constant *imposed* change in, for example, management and financial arrangements, nurse education, skill mix and in the move towards community-based child-care nursing services.

Chapman (1989) also discusses the problems of research utilisation and implementation, and suggests that research findings must be readily accessible and should be jargon-free. Jargonese is a recurring theme in the literature relating to the failure of nurses to use research in practice (Hockey, 1987; Lindeman, 1984; Fawcett, 1984). Fawcett suggests that this failure can be attributed to two sources: that is, researchers who cannot communicate in a form understandable to the average practitioner; and practitioners who do not possess sufficient understanding of the language of research to interpret research reports. Bergman (1984) discusses this issue further and places the 'blame' on publishers, who demand 'sophisticated reporting', and with the nursing education system which does not sufficiently develop the 'desire and skills' for understanding research.

McFarlane (1977) looks at the links between nursing research and nurse education, and emphasises that nursing students should be encouraged from the outset to question our 'professional wisdom and test the validity of our hypotheses about care'. Chapman (1989) discusses the need for all students of nursing to be taught to read research critically, which will enable them to see the value of a piece of research and its relevance to practice settings. Chapman suggests that this is best done by teaching critical reading skills, and by 'discussing methodologies employed, including the meanings of terms such as "significant"'. The development of such skills will enable students, and qualified practitioners, to be discerning about research findings, particularly when they are faced with conflicting data.

The Royal College of Nursing (1982) does not, however, advocate teaching research as a separate topic but suggests that it should be integrated throughout the curriculum. The English National Board (1992) has also recently adopted this approach. Certain problems exist, however, in removing research as a core theme from the nursing curriculum, not least because many nurse teachers have had little research input in their own education and many teachers lack the skills to 'integrate' research into their teaching. It is not sufficient for teachers to steer students towards available research; they must be able to evaluate critically the approach and methodology used and make judgements about validity, the appropriateness of statistical tools used, ethics, sampling methods, limitations and so on.

Another reason why nurses may be reluctant to put research into practice could be because of the failure of nurses in the past to use new knowledge effectively. A good example of this relates to midwives and the work of several psychologists about bonding. Bowlby (1965: 180) was one of the first to question the practice in the sixties of removing babies from their mothers immediately following delivery. He wrote:

let the reader reflect for a moment on the astonishing practice which has been followed in maternity wards – of separating mothers and babies immediately after birth – and ask himself whether this is a way to promote a close mother–child relationship. It is hoped that this madness of Western society will never be copied by the so-called less developed countries.

The results of these criticisms were that 'successful bonding' became such an important issue that mothers (and to some extent midwives) felt guilt and a sense of failure if complete bonding did not take place. The problem is, of course, that bonding is not something that can be measured in concrete terms. As Muller *et al.* (1992:31) discuss:

> When the theories of bonding first began to affect hospital attitudes about the early hours after delivery, there was sometimes an unfortunate effect from overstating the significance of early intervention, which consequently led to parents feeling guilty, or failures, if something prevented them from making the appropriate overtures to their infant. Previous experience, home background as well as beliefs and attitudes all contribute to the complexity of factors which can exert effects on early parent–infant interaction.

A further explanation for not utilising research stems from the many medical research reports which offer conflicting views on the same subject. Frequently, when teaching child-care nurses about research, they cite conflicting research findings about, for example, infant feeding and diet. The result of such conflict may result in nurses failing to utilise any research in their practice, possibly because of a fear that they may be wrong. Yet, if nursing is to develop as a human science in its own right, nurses *must* be prepared to use their own judgement and if in doubt undertake clinical research of their own to find out for themselves which is the most effective intervention. A similar problem arises when research findings conflict with traditionally held viewpoints. An example of this inertia is the area of pain in infants. The traditionally held viewpoint was that infants were not able to feel pain because of their immature nervous systems and for a variety of other reasons. Burr (1987) discusses the lack of research into this area, particularly in relation to sick children in the community. Clearly, nurses both in hospital and in the community need to be aware of current research about the measurement and management of pain. The traditional thinking arose because infants are not able to communicate pain as adults do, and not because they are not

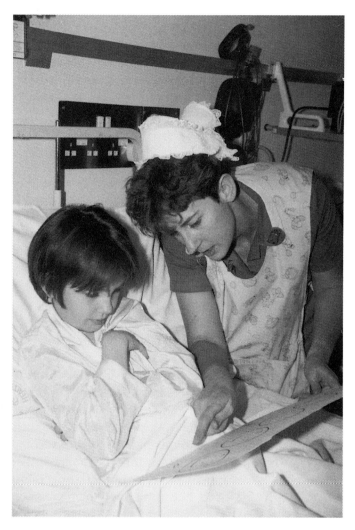

Figure 5.1 The use of pain scales can help in the assessment of pain and in evaluating the effectiveness of analgesia

experiencing pain. An excellent review of literature by Reape (1990) expels many of the myths surrounding this much neglected area of child health care.

This section has looked at why nurses fail to use research findings in their practice, and has perhaps painted a depressing picture of the reality of current nursing activity. The picture is not, however, entirely negative, and progress has been made. Indeed some child-care units are centres of excellence, and a great deal of research is used and undertaken by nurses. Unfortunately, research utilisation is not universal, and until it is we must acknowledge that not all children who are cared for by nurses are receiving the *best* care available, and our aim must be to ensure that all nurses are research-minded. Children's nurses must become more challenging of the fundamental assumptions which underpin their existing practices, thus creating an awareness of the future needs of both children and their families and of the profession.

Doing Research in Child-care Settings

So far, in this chapter, the emphasis has been placed on using findings from nursing and psychological research. We move now to look at the need for nurses to undertake clinical research in child-care settings so that they can add to the body of nursing knowledge in the field of child health care.

Nursing research is the systematic and scientific investigation of phenomena in order to update or add to the existing body of nursing knowledge. In child care, as in other disciplines, there is a need for a variety of philosophical approaches to research. In many instances, the knowledge available about specific aspects of child care is so sparse that a phenomenological approach is desirable in order to explore aspects of care and to generate new theory. In other cases, it involves nurses having a knowledge of relevant past research so that they can build on, and progress from, existing knowledge, by the further development and testing of theory.

It is important that a forward momentum be achieved, with child-care nurses continually updating their practice through research. If this fails to happen then we are in danger as a profession of working from a consistently out-of-date knowledge base, of not being able effectively to adapt to change or keep pace with colleagues from other related disciplines. Ultimately, if nursing is to evolve as a discipline distinct from other disciplines it must demonstrate the research base of its practice.

Although this section is not intended as a practical guide to understanding research (there are many good books which can assist nurses to develop essential research skills, some of which are included in the Reference section at the end of this chapter), it does seek to explore some of the fundamental considerations of undertaking research in child health – such as who should undertake research, what problems they should address, how they should approach those problems and finally, what are the specific difficulties of undertaking research with children.

Much of the existing research base of child-care nursing has been derived from the work of sociologists, doctors and psychologists. Although there does exist a pool of research-based knowledge derived from nursing research, a great deal of this research has tended to be undertaken by nurses enrolled on certificate- and diploma-level nursing courses, who have frequently been restricted in what they have studied, because of the limitations of time and money, and in how they have studied, because of the tradition of academic institutions to favour quantitative approaches. Other limitations, such as a lack of access to research subjects and inadequate resources to travel further than the immediate vicinity, have resulted in small-scale quantitative studies, small samples and, in some cases, doubtful data-collection instruments, resulting in what can only be described as suspect internal and external validity.

This research, done for the sake of 'doing' research, may well use the sophisticated language and jargon required by educational institutions, but often lacks depth. Fortunately, most colleges of nursing, institutions of further and higher education and universities are now discouraging students, apart from those on graduate, post-graduate and doctoral courses, from undertaking research and have concentrated more on ensuring that nurses are able, to critically evaluate previously published research. Colleges and universities are also becoming more flexible in accepting phenomenological approaches to research undertaken by those nurses on post-graduate nursing programmes, although Robinson (1992) suggests that the major funding bodies for nursing research are still not entirely happy about these unpositivistic approaches.

So who are the nurse researchers of the future? Nursing research should without doubt be undertaken by nurses (Moody, 1990), and child-care nursing research should be undertaken by those nurses who work with children. One way of ensuring that nurses have the opportunity to undertake research in their area of practice is to encourage nurses to undertake post-registration study to degree level or higher. This involves allowing nurses study time and ensuring that funding is available for professional development. Unfortunately, in the present financial climate of the health service, such opportunities are liable to be limited, although the

United Kingdom Central Council and English National Board initiatives, such as the Higher Award, may well enhance post-registration educational opportunities for many.

A second option is to assist qualified nurses to undertake research courses as part of their in-service development and encourage them to undertake research in their practice settings. It is encouraging that the English National Board, by making research one of the key characteristics of the Higher Award, has recognised the need for nurses to develop research skills. It is worth mentioning here that research nurses, employed by many health authorities, can be a valuable source of information and facilitate such research activities, by advising about problem identification, appropriate ways of studying particular problems, data collection and analysis. Such experienced researchers can help to prevent the novice researcher from making common errors, as well as being a useful resource.

Thirdly, nurses can find out for themselves how to undertake research by studying methodology and by keeping up to date with current research and developments in their field of practice. Nurses need to adopt a questioning approach to their work in order to identify researchable problems from practice and develop appropriate skills for problem solving through research. This does not necessarily involve nurses designing complex methodologies. Replicating appropriate research, for example, enables nurses to solve problems without having to design intricate sampling strategies or data collection instruments and can be useful in updating knowledge.

Finally, collaboration with other disciplines or with professional researchers from within nursing can be helpful in the search for knowledge. In child care, as in other spheres of nursing, nurses do not work in isolation from other professionals, and problems are often multifactorial in nature. It is therefore often appropriate for nurses to 'team up' with professionals from other disciplines in order to investigate problems from a broader stance.

What research should be undertaken?

Nursing is essentially a practice discipline, and there is undoubtedly a need for research which addresses significant problems arising from clinical practice that can add to the body of nursing knowledge and be utilised by nurses in their practice. This is not meant to imply that research should concentrate on physiological aspects of care, but that nurses should identify and investigate problems relating to the holistic needs of the child and family. It is important that research is not undertaken haphazardly or in isolation, but that it builds on previous knowledge so that it can further develop the knowledge bases of practice. There are vast areas of child-care practice that are under-researched, or where change has rendered previous research out of date, or where research from other disciplines, particularly medicine and pharmacology, have advanced knowledge and technology, but there is an insufficient nursing knowledge base which can adequately guide nursing practice.

It often seems that there is such a dearth of children's nursing research that it is sometimes difficult to prioritise research activities so that really significant problems are investigated. It is interesting to note that Brown *et al.* (1984), in a review of American nursing research undertaken during the 1970s, showed that less than a third of nursing published research was of use to practice. It is important that we do not fall into the trap of undertaking research for its own sake. Resources, both human and financial, are likely to be far too scarce in the 1990s for the mistakes of the last decades to be repeated.

Identifying exactly what research should be undertaken relies heavily on our ability to ask important questions about our practice. Moody (1990) suggests that the development of a research question involves creativity, imagination, ingenuity, interest and commitment. Thus in child care it requires that practitioners be observant and reflective in their practice and take time to identify which important issues need investigating and then spend further time and energy in refining research problems into researchable questions. In practical terms, the problems that arise from nursing children today can be succinctly categorised under six main headings:

1 *Problems emanating from changes in the structure and organisation of nursing care.* For example, what will be the effects of reducing the qualified/unqualified ratio of nursing staff in acute and chronic child care settings? Is primary nursing effective in acute children's wards?

2 *Problems arising from governmental legislation.* For example, what is the effect of general practitioner fundholding upon children with chronic ill health? What implications in practice will the 1989 Children Act have on children with learning disabilities?

3 *Problems arising from advances in technical and other scientific knowledge.* For example, what are the most appropriate nursing interventions for nursing children undergoing chemotherapy for clinical AIDS? What are the most effective techniques available to nurses involved in teaching parents to care for ventilator-dependent babies at home?

4 *Problems arising from national and local guidelines.* For example, how can nurses in the accident and emergency department ensure that children receive the services recommended by the Department of Health (1991) in *The Welfare of Children and Young People in Hospital*? How can nurses help parents who wish to accompany their children to the anaesthetic room prior to surgery?

5 *Problems arising from existing nursing knowledge.* For example, what are the implications of the research by Mayall (1991) which shows that mothers and health visitors have widely different perspectives on child care? What are the implications of research by Kitzinger (1991) which explores the role of mothers in child sexual abuse?

6 *Problems arising from a lack of knowledge about phenomena.* For example, how do terminally ill children wish to spend their remaining time? Do children in intensive care benefit from play therapy?

Defining and refining a problem statement is not easy, but it is essential if nurses are to engage in research successfully. The refinement stage should lead the nurse researcher comfortably to identifying researchable questions and thus deciding upon a conceptual schema for studying the problem. Three levels of research question can be used in child-care research. Level one questions are *exploratory or descriptive*, and address a single concept and usually refer to one study population, where there is little or no existing available knowledge about the concept. An example of a level one question might be 'What are the psychological and social needs of sick children and their families in the community?'. This type of question is appropriate here because previous knowledge about the specific needs of sick children in the community, who would have traditionally been hospitalised, is limited.

Level two questions are *correlational* questions, which often develop as a result of exploratory or descriptive research, where some knowledge about the variables which relate to a concept is known. These questions will explore the relationship between two or more variables, for example, what is the relationship between the proposed career choice of adolescent girls and anorexia nervosa?'

Level three questions are *explanatory/predictive*-type questions, which build on exploratory and correlational research, aiming to identify, or make predictions about, causal relationships between two or more variables. An example of this type of question would be 'Why does fluid restriction in children post tonsillectomy result in a higher incidence of haemorrhage?'.

How can children's nurses undertake research?

The way in which nurses decide to approach research must ultimately stem from the nature of the problem and the research question(s). However, nurses have in the past tended to be influenced by the 'fashion' of the day. The problem is that in many cases questions from practice which should have been studied from one philosophical stance have been manipulated so that they could be studied from an alternative stance. For example, a problem which should have been thoroughly explored inductively because little previous work had been undertaken, is investigated deductively in spite of a lack of available theory upon which to base the investigation or sufficient knowledge of important variables. The preoccupation of many of these earlier nursing researchers stemmed from the belief that if nursing research was to be 'respectable' then the positivistic approach had to be used (Robinson, 1992). Leininger (1985) goes so far as to suggest that this over-concentration upon scientific approaches as the only source of nursing knowledge has been responsible for the 'limited substantive knowledge about the nature of nursing'. Child-care research has been a predictable casualty of nurses' need to be perceived as natural and 'respectable' scientists, as the dearth of substantial qualitative studies undertaken during the 1970s and 1980s will testify. Over the last decade, nurses fortunately seem to have lost this need to satisfy other professionals from the natural sciences and have moved away from this positivistic stance, to the extent where much more nursing research is now qualitative in approach, using phenomenological and ethnographic methods. This shift was perhaps inevitable, with the current emphasis on holistic, family-centred care rather than the pragmatic, mechanistic and reductionistic approaches to care employed in the past. It must be said, however, that in child-care research we must be careful to learn from the mistakes of the past and not over-concentrate on any one approach. By the very nature of the problems facing nurses working with children in various settings, there will be a need to engage in multiple approaches in the pursuit of knowledge.

The choice of data-collection instruments must then largely rely on the problem and the research question(s). If questions are exploratory in nature, then observational methods, open-ended questionnaires and unstructured interviews are usually the methods of choice. Correlational and predictive questions, because they rely heavily on the identification and control of variables and tend to use statistical analysis, require much more precise data, which can easily and effectively be quantified. Methods of choice are those which will yield such data – for example, biophysical measurements, structured questionnaires and structured interviews. In child-care research, however, the use of some data-collection instrumentation is limited because of the child's age, cognitive development, language skills, experience and intellect. These issues will be further explored later on.

Problems in undertaking research on children

The ethical implications of undertaking research with any human subjects are always complex and profound. The dividing line between appropriate research and unethical treatment of subjects is frequently unclear (Oyster *et al.*, 1987). The ethical issues involved with undertaking research with children are further complicated in distinct areas: informed consent, therapeutic clinical research, and non-therapeutic clinical research.

The 1961 Declaration of Helsinki states that clinical research on human subjects cannot be undertaken without free consent after the subject has been informed and, *if legally incompetent*, without the consent of the legal guardian. The arguments in relation to children revolve around the extent to which children are able to give this *free consent*, and whether consent by parents or guardians is really ethical or is merely obtained to protect the doctor or institution from litigation (Thompson *et al.*, 1988). Ramsey (1976, 1977) argues that a child's lack of knowledge and cognition about either medicine or the legal implications of consent invalidates any attempts to obtain free consent which is truly informed. McCormack (1976), on the other hand, argues that children should participate in both therapeutic and non-therapeutic clinical research as long as there is no more than minimal or negligible risk to the child, if the research is scientifically designed and if there is consent by proxy. Beauchamp and Childress (1983) suggest that McCormack sees the participation of children (and adults) in research as a matter of justice; that is, that we should bear certain burdens for the common good of all.

The issue of informed consent in children is further complicated by attempts to specify the age at which children are able to consent to participate in research of their own volition – in other words, when children are able to make informed consent. It is evident that the ability to consent involves the cognitive and moral development of the child. Making judgements about the child's ability involves, to some extent, the subjective judgement of the person seeking consent. The issue is further complicated by the type of research being undertaken; that is, whether the research is therapeutic or non-therapeutic. Therapeutic research – that is, research which is related to the child's health status and which may benefit the child directly – is generally thought to be more acceptable as long as certain principles are adhered to and ethical codes are not broken. Such principles include the significance of the problem to be researched, the nature of the information sought and what the child is required to do to yield that information, and whether the benefits of the research outweigh the risks involved to the child. The extent to which these principles are considered again depends to some extent on the subjectivity of the researcher and the difficulties of an adult ever being able to view the world from the perspective of a child.

The issue of undertaking non-therapeutic research on children is even more complex and has been the subject of much debate. Non-therapeutic research is research undertaken usually on healthy subjects, which will not benefit the subject but which may benefit society as a whole. An example of such research was the Willowbrook hepatitis experiment (see Beauchamp and Childress, 1983). Willowbrook, an institution for children with learning disabilities in New York, had a high incidence of hepatitis, albeit a mild strain. Several studies were undertaken at Willowbrook in the late 1950s and early 1960s, including some which involved exposing healthy children to hepatitis in an attempt to find a vaccination against the disease. The dilemma here is that the children were healthy but were at risk because nearly all children admitted to the institution developed hepatitis within the first year and that the research was justifiable because of beneficence to future generations. Whether children should be used in non-therapeutic research for whatever reason has been strongly attacked by Ramsey (1976, 1977), on the grounds that they cannot give free consent and thus their integrity is violated. McCormack (1976) takes an opposing view, that if the risks are negligible, if consent is given by the guardian of the child and if the research is scientifically sound, then using children in non-therapeutic research can be justifiable for the common good of all. The complexity of these opposing views confounds the issue of non-therapeutic research to the extent that it remains unclear as to what is, and what is not, permissible. The general opinion, according to Brykczynska (1989), is that unless a child can consent to participation, non-therapeutic and invasive research should not be conducted.

Nurses should not consider themselves immune to ethical debate and principles because they perceive them to be relevant only to medical research involving invasive procedures or pharmaceutics. Although most nursing research involving children does not involve subjecting them to physical harm, nurses must consider the psychological and emotional effects of their actions, the potential loss of trust and the potential generation of anxiety in participants (Holm and Llewellyn, 1986). Clearly, too, nurses have a duty to children in their care who are participating in other research, apart from nursing research. Nurses are often in a position of *knowing* their patients and having a deeper relationship with them, than would a researcher from an alternative discipline. Thus the nurse may be the only person to notice signs of anxiety or stress in the child participating in research. As with any research subject, the child has the right to withdraw from participation, and the nurse should ensure that they are permitted to withdraw without pressure from the researcher to continue being involved.

A second problem of undertaking research on children involves data-collection techniques. Studies which involve observation or self-reporting instruments (questionnaires, interviews) may present problems to researchers. Observational studies were popular during the 1970s and 1980s (Moody, 1990), with over 50 per cent of nursing studies in the United States during these years being observational. Ethically, overt observation is easier to justify than covert observation, but researchers have to account for *reactivity* as a potential threat to internal validity (reactivity refers to research subjects changing their behaviours because they are being studied, rather than in response to an imposed manipulation). In research with adults, researchers have used covert participant observation as a way of controlling reactivity, or, when undertaking research with children in educational settings, have participated in the culture of a school so that children under study view them as part of the organisation rather than as an outsider. This technique can be employed by nurse researchers in settings where children are used to seeing nurses and interacting with them. The issue of obtaining informed consent in this type of research is evident, and researchers must be able to justify the covert nature of their study.

Designing self-reporting instruments for use in research with children can also be problematic. Oyster *et al.* (1987) discuss the necessity of ensuring that the wording used in interviews and questionnaires does not become a barrier to subjects responding to questions. For example, if asking a 3-year-old child about the nature and location of pain, words such as 'intensity' or 'acute' would certainly be inappropriate. It is important, then, that in designing tools for data collection with child subjects, these tools are sensitive to the age, understanding and cognition of the child. As with any research using such instruments, care must be taken by the researcher to ensure the reliability of tools. The many pain scales that have been designed for use with children are a good example of child-sensitive tools which have been adequately tested for reliability and validity (see Alder, 1991).

Conclusions

Research-mindedness is an important characteristic of professional nursing in the contemporary health services. Nurses, regardless of the speciality in which they practise, must develop the skills and knowledge needed to use and undertake research in order to expand the knowledge base of the profession and ensure that the care delivered is effective and sound.

The dearth of research into the care of children leaves a place for both qualitative and quantitative approaches to the study of significant problems. The changing nature of child-care nursing will require that both approaches are appropriate for many years to come. Nurses working in child care do, however, face unique problems when undertaking research, particularly in relation to ethical considerations and the collection of data. These problems are apparent regardless of the approach researchers take when addressing important research questions. Researchers who are experienced in identifying significant problems and in formulating researchable questions find that usually the design and data-collection methods are evident. Researchers wishing to undertake research on child subjects may find that, although methodologies may be evident, the nature of their subjects restricts how they go about answering research questions.

References

Alder, S. (1991) 'Taking children at their word: pain control in paediatrics'. In Glasper, A. (ed.) *Child Care: Some Nursing Perspectives*. London: Wolfe.

Beauchamp, T. and Childress, J. (1983) *Principles of Biomedical Ethics*, 2nd edn, New York: Oxford University Press.

Bergman, R. (1984) 'Omissions in nursing research', *International Nursing Review*, 31(2): 55–6.

Bowlby, J. (1953) *Child Care and the Growth of Love*, Harmondsworth: Penguin.

Bowlby, J. (1965) *Child Care and the Growth of Love*, revised edn, Harmondsworth: Penguin.

Breu, C. and Dracup, K. (1976) 'Implementing nursing research in a critical care setting', *Journal of Nursing Administration*, 6(10): 14–17.

Brown, J. S., Tanner, C. A. and Padrick, K. P. (1984) 'Nursing's search for scientific knowledge', *Nursing Research*, 33: 26–32.

Brown, R. (1989) *Individualised Care*, Middlesex: Scutari Press.

Brykczynska, G. (ed.) (1989) *Ethics in Paediatric Nursing*, London: Chapman and Hall.

Burr, S. (1987) 'Pain in childhood', *Nursing*, Series 3(24): 890–5.

Chapman, C. (1989) 'Research for action: the way forward', *Senior Nurse*, 9(6): 17–18.

Cleary, J. (1977) 'The distribution of nursing attention in a children's ward', *Nursing Times*, 73: 93–8.

Consumers' Association (1985) *Children in Hospital*, London: Consumers' Association.

Declaration of Helsinki (1961) The World Medical Association.

Department of Health (1989) *The Children Act*, London: HMSO.

Department of Health (1991) *The Welfare of Children and Young People in Hospital*, London: HMSO.

English National Board (1992) Circular 1992/09/RLV, 'Additional guidelines for the development of pre-registration courses leading to parts 12–15 of the Professional Register and the Dip H.E.', London: ENB.

Fawcett, J. (1984) 'Another look at utilisation of nursing research', *The Journal of Nursing Scholarship*, XVI(2): 59–60.

Harris, P. (1979) 'Children, their parents and hospital', University of Nottingham, Unpublished PhD thesis.

Hawthorn, P. (1975) *Nurse, I Want My Mummy!*, London: RCN.

Hockey, L. (1987) 'Issues in the communication of nursing research', *Recent Advances in Nursing*, 18: 154–67.

Holm, K. and Llewellyn, J. G. (1986) *Nursing Research for Nursing Practice*, Philadelphia: W. B. Saunders.

Hunt, J. (1981) 'Indicators for nursing practice: the use of research findings', *Journal of Advanced Nursing*, 6: 189–194.

Kitzinger, J. (1991) 'Child sexual abuse and the trials of motherhood', in S. Wyke and J. Hewison (eds) *Child Health Matters*, Milton Keynes: Open University Press.

Leininger, M. M. (ed.) (1985) *Qualitative Research Methods in Nursing*, Orlando, FL: Grune and Stratton.

Lindeman, C. A. (1984) 'Dissemination of nursing research', *The Journal of Nursing Scholarship*, XVI(2): 57–8.

Lovely, E. M. (1951) *The Nursing of Sick Children*, Edinburgh: E. and S. Livingstone.

Lynn, M. R. (1989) 'Research in practice: no individual's responsibility', *Journal of Paediatric Nursing*, 4(5): 374–6.

McCormack, R. (1976) 'Experiments in children: sharing sociality', *Hastings Center Report No. 6*, pp. 41–46.

McFarlane, J. K. (1977) 'Developing a theory of nursing: the relation of theory to practice, education and research', *Journal of Advanced Nursing*, 2: 261–70.

Mayall, B. (1991) 'Ideologies of child care: mothers and health visitors', in S. Wyke and J. Hewison (eds) *Child Health Matters*, Milton Keynes: Open University Press.

Moody, L. (1990) *Advancing Nursing Science through Theory*, vols I and II, Newbury Park, CA: Sage.

Muller, D. J., Harris, P. J., Wattley, L. and Taylor, J. (1992) *Nursing Children: Psychology, Research and Practice*, 2nd edn, London: Chapman and Hall.

Myers, B. (1910) *The Care of Children*, London: Henry Kimpton.

Oyster, C. K., Hanten, W. P. and Llorens, L. A. (1987) *Introduction to Research: a Guide for the Health Science Professional*, Philadelphia: Lippincott.

Pearce, E. (1938) *A Short Encyclopaedia for Nurses*, 3rd edn, London: Faber and Faber.

Platt, H. (1959) *The Welfare of Children in Hospital: Report of the Committee on Child Health Services*, London: HMSO.

Poster, E. C. (1983) 'Stress immunization: techniques to help children cope with hospitalization', *Maternal-Child Nursing Journal*, 12: 119–34.

Ramsey, P. (1976) 'The enforcement of morals: non-therapeutic research on children', *Hastings Center Report No. 6*, pp. 29–31.

Ramsey, P. (1977) 'Children as research subjects', *Hastings Center Report No. 7*, pp. 40–42.

Reape, D. (1990) 'Children and pain', *Nursing Standard*, 4(16): 33–6.

Robertson, J. and Robertson, J. (1989) *Separation and the Very Young*, London: Free Association Press.

Robinson, K. (1992) 'The real world of research', Part 1, *Nursing Times Special Supplement*, 88: 43.

Rodin, J. (1983) *Will This Hurt?*, London: RCN.

Royal College of Nursing (1982) *Research-mindedness and Nurse Education*, London: RCN.

Thompson, I. E., Melia, K. M. and Boyd, M. (1988) *Nursing Ethics*, 2nd edn, London: Churchill Livingstone.

Weller, B. (1980) *Helping Sick Children Play*, London: Baillière Tindall.

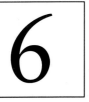

CULTURAL ASPECTS OF CHILDREN'S HEALTH AND ILLNESS

Barbara F. Weller
Independent Nurse Consultant

In 1990 there were more than $2\frac{1}{2}$ million people living in the United Kingdom whose ethnic origins were from what has been described as the New Commonwealth. Together with migrants from the Irish Republic and Europe, they comprise about 10 per cent of the total population (OPCS, 1990). Although there have been well-established but small ethnic minority groups in the United Kingdom for many generations, our society has only relatively recently – within the past few decades or so – become truly multicultural. Then the flourishing economy of the 1950s and 1960s encouraged migration to the British Isles. That we now share in the United Kingdom a variety of cultural heritages is true for the children and their families, and also for professionals working within the health services.

More recently the United Kingdom has seen the arrival of smaller groups of refugees, usually in a response to the political situation in their own country, posing special and distinct problems for the children of these families. Eisenbruch (1988) suggests that these children may experience a powerful grief reaction, not only in response to the personal loss of loved ones, but also to the loss of their culture. Personal bereavement and cultural bereavement are complementary, and early losses of family and culture can seed problems for children and young people which can emerge even after apparent satisfactory resettlement of the family.

Most of the ethnic minority population in the United Kingdom is concentrated in deprived inner-city areas, where they share the same social class disadvantages as other residents: those of poor housing and educational facilities, low income and lack of employment opportunities with the consequent implications for the health of the individual families (Mares *et al.*,

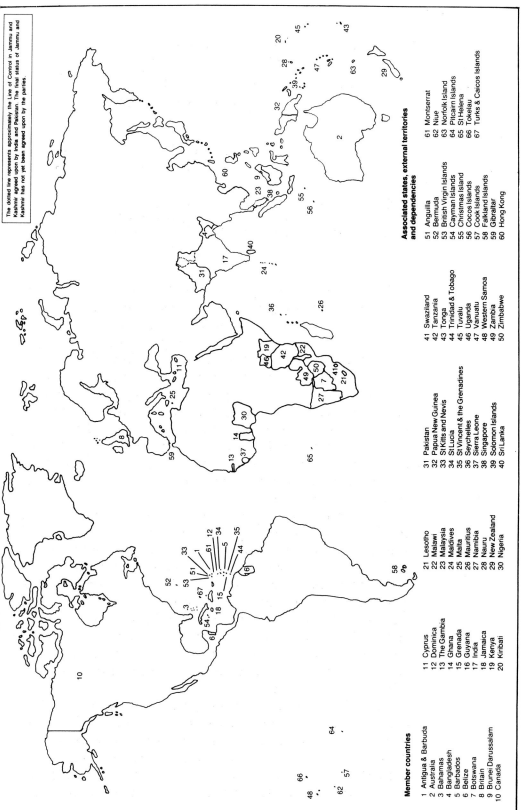

The dotted line represents approximately the Line of Control in Jammu and Kashmir agreed upon by India and Pakistan. The final status of Jammu and Kashmir has not yet been agreed upon by the parties.

Member countries

1 Antigua & Barbuda
2 Australia
3 Bahamas
4 Bangladesh
5 Barbados
6 Belize
7 Botswana
8 Britain
9 Brunei Darussalam
10 Canada

11 Cyprus
12 Dominica
13 The Gambia
14 Ghana
15 Grenada
16 Guyana
17 India
18 Jamaica
19 Kenya
20 Kiribati

21 Lesotho
22 Malawi
23 Malaysia
24 Maldives
25 Malta
26 Mauritius
27 Namibia
28 Nauru
29 New Zealand
30 Nigeria

31 Pakistan
32 Papua New Guinea
33 St Kitts and Nevis
34 St Lucia
35 St Vincent & the Grenadines
36 Seychelles
37 Sierra Leone
38 Singapore
39 Solomon Islands
40 Sri Lanka

41 Swaziland
42 Tanzania
43 Tonga
44 Trinidad & Tobago
45 Tuvalu
46 Uganda
47 Vanuatu
48 Western Samoa
49 Zambia
50 Zimbabwe

Associated states, external territories and dependencies

51 Anguilla
52 Bermuda
53 British Virgin Islands
54 Cayman Islands
55 Christmas Island
56 Cocos Islands
57 Cook Islands
58 Falkland Islands
59 Gibraltar
60 Hong Kong

61 Montserrat
62 Niue
63 Norfolk Island
64 Pitcairn Islands
65 St Helena
66 Tokelau
67 Turks & Caicos Islands

Figure 6.1 The New Commonwealth

1985). People from black ethnic minorities suffer a further disadvantage as they may also be subject to overt racism in their face-to-face encounters with the indigenous white population.

Kareem and Littlewood (1992) report that although there is little statistical information about the general psychological adjustment of black people, ample evidence has now been accumulated which shows that to be black in Britain today is to be exposed to a variety of adverse stimuli which can have a detrimental effect on mental health.

Culture

There are probably as many definitions of culture as there are different cultures in the world. A useful definition is one provided by Linton (1940), who suggested that culture was 'the sum total of knowledge, attitudes and habitual behaviour patterns shared and transmitted by the members of a particular society'.

'Culture' is therefore the learned, socially acquired traditions and life styles of the members of a society or of a family, including their patterned, repetitive ways of thinking, feeling, acting and behaving. Cultural diversity accounts for variations in family life and relationships, food preferences, religious beliefs, communication modes and values. Culture is probably the most important part of the human environment because it defines the way of life for a particular group of people.

Cultural beliefs therefore form the basis for the main aspects of people's lives, including child-rearing or parenting practices and child health care. The continuity of cultural values and traditions does not depend upon particular individuals. But children, as members of a family and a society, initially learn the attributes of their particular culture from parents and relatives and then later from other members of their society.

Although the culture of a particular society tends to be similar in many respects from one generation to the next, culture is not a static, fixed entity but modifies with time and adapts also to changes in the society from which it arises. Asian children, for example, brought up in a 'Western' culture may develop a taste for chips and tomato sauce because this is something they have learned from peers to enjoy. This process has been described as 'acculturation' or the adoption of host culture practices, which may not always be acceptable to the parents or traditional elders in the ethnic community and may become a cause of family stress and misunderstanding. Niederhauser

(1989) emphasises the need for sensitivity when working with second- and third-generation immigrants, where conflicts may arise in the family dynamics when traditional rituals and practices passed down from immigrant elders conflict with current health-care practices or social situations.

Some cultural practices are obvious – for example the wearing of the shalwar kameez or of a kilt – but other aspects of culture are not so immediately identifiable. Racial stereotypes can be applied to individuals or to groups. Johnson (1986) asserts that racial stereotypes of black families are very much in evidence amongst health-care professionals, illustrating this with quotations such as 'Asian women keep to themselves' and 'West Indians believe in firm discipline administered in the home'. Stereotyping from dress, skin colour or religious denomination is to make assumptions about a child or person that may prove false – not all men wearing kilts are Scots!

There is a rich diversity in any social group of attitudes, health beliefs, expectations and behaviour. The fact that such variations are less than obvious to the health-care provider makes it important for the nurse to question assumptions and to seek appropriate information from the parents and, where possible, the child.

Equally important is the recognition by the nurse of the influence of cultural beliefs and values on professional practice, assessment and intervention. The work of Davitz and Davitz (1985) clearly shows how the nurse's assessment of the patient's pain and suffering often failed to take account of cultural differences in acceptable external behaviour in the expression of pain. This frequently led to inadequate analgesia being given for pain relief.

It is perhaps a cliché, but nevertheless true, that the child's family does not have to be foreign-born to be foreign to the nurse's way. Nurses have their own subculture, defined not by ethnicity or race but by training and socialisation into a profession with its own values, rituals and belief systems.

The importance of avoiding stereotyping and ethnic generalisations in day-to-day care by any health-care worker cannot be over-emphasised. Stereotyping leads to relating to people in fixed ways and reducing the parent's and child's opportunities for access to health information. Consequently, this limits the family's choice in the adoption of new practices towards health promotion or in the understanding of treatment.

Barn's review (1990) of black children in local authority care showed that whereas black children are more likely to enter care on a voluntary basis, for reasons such as family relationships and socio-economic conditions, white children are more likely to enter care on a compulsory basis, for reasons such as parental neglect/inadequacy, delinquency, non-school attendance and child abuse. The reasons for the different patterns of referral to 'care' were explained in terms of social workers' perceptions of individual cases.

Other workers, Cameron *et al.* (1988), also found support for this premise, in that the stereotyping of clients/patients from ethnic minority groups affected the health-care worker's view of their clients'/patients' health needs and influenced the appropriateness of professional interventions.

Assessing the health-care needs of children from diverse cultural backgrounds can be difficult, especially when language barriers are present and there is a lack of understanding by health-care workers of varying cultural practices. But nursing staff need to be aware and sensitive to the richness and diversity of cultural influences and how these affect the way a family may perceive, experience and cope with their child's illness. A knowledge of and a sensitivity to the cultural beliefs of the child's family will assist the nurse in understanding behaviours that may seem at first negative, confusing or illogical, and help in producing a therapeutic response that is more appropriate for the child's condition (Brunner and Suddarth, 1991).

Leininger (1981), an American nurse anthropologist, suggests that a major challenge for all health personnel in the delivery of health-care services is to examine their own practices of ethnocentrism, cultural imposition, exclusion and accommodation in education and health-service practices.

Our predominantly ethnocentric pattern of health-care provision in the NHS has not essentially shifted since its inception in 1948, when the service was established to meet the needs of a fairly homogeneous British culture. The current pattern of health-care provision is essentially geared to life styles, family patterns, dietary habits and religious beliefs which may be neither acceptable to nor understood by many families needing health care for their children. Ethnocentrism refers to the belief that the values and practices of one culture are superior to and of greater worth than those of an alternative culture (Thiederman, 1986), based on the assumption that one's own ways of doing things are the best ways or even the only way to do them! This can lead to cultural imposition – where one's own values may be imposed upon the child and their family regardless of their beliefs and ideas.

Cultural exclusion refers to the conscious or unconscious avoidance, or omission, of cultural values and practices in planning and providing for health care or in health promotion. This can be identified in professional practice in a variety of ways, such as placing non-English-speaking people at the end of a clinic or excluding people from reports and other activities because 'they would not understand' or that 'they are too difficult to work with'. 'Unreachable', 'unmotivated' and 'resistant' are all labels that have been applied to patients, families or clients who are perceived to be 'difficult' or 'awkward' by health-care professionals who also fail to realise that these are terms that may equally apply to themselves. They may not understand what is being said to them, or if they do, may not want to hear it (Zola, 1973).

Healing Systems

Most communities, even those in the developed world, provide a pluralist system of health care and treatment including traditional healers in their healing systems: a mixture of sacred and secular (Helman, 1990), alongside biomedical practitioners.

Kleinman (1980) has suggested that there are three overlapping sectors of health care: the popular sector, the folk sector and the professional sector – a hierarchy of resort. Each sector has its own code, defining who is the healer and who is the patient and their interaction in the therapeutic encounter.

The popular sector

This is the lay sector of health care where 'illness' is first defined or diagnosed. Treatments may be suggested or given by family members, neighbours or work colleagues; that is, people with whom there is usually already a link of friendship or kinship. No payment is made for the advice or remedy. It has been estimated that between 70 and 90 per cent of all health care takes place within this sector, in both Western and non-Western societies (Helman, 1990).

The folk sector

An awareness of the beliefs of the popular (family, community), and folk (non-professional healers) domains of health care available to a particular family is important. This is helpful to the nurse in promoting compliances and co-operation in treatment and care, as issues can be discussed as they arise and any discrepancies resolved.

In the United Kingdom there has been a growing trend in the development of supportive healing systems, including herbalism, reflexology, acupuncture, homeopathy and so on. Muslim *hakims* or Hindu *vaids*, spiritualists and faith healers too are established and may be consulted by the patients for their child alongside biomedicine, with or without the medical practitioner's knowledge.

Folk healing offers several advantages over the biomedical approach as many of these approaches involve the patient's family in the healing process. The traditional healer is most likely to hold a shared cultural view of the world with the family, unlike biomedical practitioners, who are often separated from their patients by social class, economic position, gender, specialised education and sometimes cultural background (Helman, 1990).

The professional sector

Western scientific medicine, sometimes known as biomedicine or allopathy, is, in most countries, the only medical system that is sanctioned by law. Practitioners of biomedicine include not only physicians and surgeons but also the professions auxiliary to medicine; for example nurses, midwives, radiographers or physiotherapists. Medical practitioners enjoy positions of high social status, higher incomes and more clearly defined rights and obligations than other types of healers. They have considerable power to prescribe drugs and treatments and in some instances to deprive people of their freedom by confining them to hospital (Helman, 1990).

Like its clients and patients, the scientific medical system is not insulated from cultural influences. Payer (1990), examining the medical systems of the United States, Germany, France and the United Kingdom, identified national differences in diagnostic categories and noted that certain medical beliefs, treatments and practices are influenced by the core, dominant cultural values in each of these societies.

The hospital provides the main focus for the delivery of biomedical treatment to which the general practitioner in the community will commonly refer. This is in contrast to the folk and popular sectors, where the patient remains at home amongst family and friends.

Therapeutic networking ⎯⎯⎯⎯⎯⎯⎯⎯⎯⎯⎯⎯⎯⎯⎯⎯⎯⎯⎯

Although the 'hierarchy of resort' relating the three sectors of health care has been identified, the family may move in and out of each sector. At times it may span all three, taking advice and information from one to the other to use as considered appropriate for their 'sick' child. Indeed, some traditional healers in the United Kingdom advise their clients to consult the family's biomedical practitioner for access to investigative screening, such as to confirm haemoglobin levels.

Early Parenting Practices ⎯⎯⎯⎯⎯⎯⎯⎯⎯⎯⎯⎯⎯⎯⎯⎯

Beliefs about child rearing are usually bound up with beliefs about life itself. They are culturally transmitted and culturally learned. They are also held without question. Beliefs and values will differ from group to group, and what is regarded as good and bad behaviour. Other cultural variations affecting child-rearing practices will include who does the teaching and how it is done; the age at which the child is expected to achieve certain types of behaviour or learning; the support given to children while they are growing up and by whom; and the cultural core values about what is important in life to inculcate in children (for example, in many cultures respect for elders is carefully taught). In all societies, pregnancy and childbirth are more than physiological events: they are recognised also as social events of significance for the woman, her partner and the family as well. The process of attachment or bonding of a mother to her infant, the foundation of parenting, includes pregnancy, giving birth, seeing the baby, touching the baby and care-taking (Johnston, 1980). It is the way in which this process is carried out that will be defined by the norms or rules in each society and may vary within a particular society.

During childbirth the conditions and techniques for giving birth are various. In some societies the primiparous woman is expected to return to her parent's home to give birth. In these societies, older women are nearby to provide support and counsel on how to nurse, how to cope with the infant's crying and with general care. There is a strong belief that the labouring woman should not be cared for in a strange hospital by an unknown male doctor but rather that she should stay where she is known and loved. The actual process of delivery, cord care and placenta disposal is carried out by a female traditional birth attendant who is known to the community.

The majority of women in the United Kingdom do not follow these practices: most confinements take place in hospital. But the importance of recognising and facilitating traditional practices during this time are important for the future well-being of the child and mother. It may, for example, be more appropriate for the labouring woman to have as her companion her mother or mother-in-law rather than her husband or partner, now the common practice in our society. Occasionally, Asian Muslim parents may ask for the placenta so that they can bury it, as they may find it offensive for it to be incinerated or otherwise disposed of.

Infant feeding and weaning practices, too, vary enormously; for example, some mothers consider that the giving of colostrum to the newborn infant is unhealthy as it is unclean, like pus, or simply not real milk, appearing as it does thin and pale compared to mature breast milk. Instead, some mothers may offer substitute liquids such as water flavoured with sugar, anise or herbs for the first feeds. Ahmet (1990) cites an example on one post-natal ward where Sylheti mothers from Bangladesh were expressing and discarding litres of colostrum unknown to the midwives because of these beliefs.

Breast feeding is the norm in many societies and highly regarded by many religions. Bohay's study (1991), amongst Ukrainian (second- and third-generation) mothers living in the United States revealed that breast feeding held a strong health value in the Ukrainian culture, for the new-born and infant: 'being healthy is being breastfed'. For the mother, breast feeding contributed to her cultural and emotional well-being. 'The mothers shall give suck to their offspring for two whole years' Quran (or Koran), the Muslim Holy Book. However, in the West, where a safe, cheap alternative is available, many mothers choose the method of bottle feeding with an infant food formula. Dobson (1991) reported from her study amongst Punjabi women living in England that over half of the mothers interviewed breast fed initially but had commenced bottle feeding by eight weeks postpartum. A number of other studies of immigrant mothers confirm a similar trend of the incidence of breast feeding falling from the high levels of the country of origin towards the lower levels of the inner-city communities that the mothers have joined (Ahmet, 1990).

Infant cleansing and time of the first bath are also subject to considerable variation. In some cultures the baby is ceremoniously bathed at birth and in others the vernix caseosa is allowed to remain. Some Muslims may ask for the baby to be bathed immediately after delivery in order that 'all impurities' are removed before handing over to the mother; others will accept the current hospital practice.

Evaluating Traditional Health Beliefs and Practices

Williams and Jelliffe (1972) devised an assessment system that continues to be relevant today for health-care workers to use in the evaluation of traditional health beliefs and practices. It is based on whether such practices are likely to be 'beneficial, neutral, harmful or uncertain' to the client.

A nursing assessment based on this approach to improving maternal-child health suggestions by Johnston (1980) includes an examination of the following questions:

1   *Are these practices beneficial*? What are the elements that are valuable to health in the local communities and what should be incorporated into health education? Examples of beneficial traditional child-care practices include infant massage, the early establishment of breast feeding, dietary practices that reduce sugar and salt intake.

2   *Are these practices harmless*? This would include those customs and practices that have no obvious effect on health one way or the other – although it is important to recognise that they are important to the parents and should be understood in terms of the meaning for health that these practices hold for them. The nurse's acceptance of these practices, and in some instances facilitating them, will assist in helping to put the mother at ease and in the establishment of a positive and supportive relationship. Examples would include: the wearing of amulets or charms, the ritual disposal of the placenta or culturally prescribed hygienic practices.

3   *Are these practices harmful*? These are practices that are detrimental to the health of either mother or child, and should be modified. Examples would include: extreme forms of slimming diets, the avoidance of giving colostrum to the new-born infant, the applications of surma containing lead to the child's or breast-feeding woman's eyelids to make them look big and bright.

4   *Are these practices uncertain*? Some traditional practices are difficult to classify. These may include the use of diets and herbal remedies or the presence of siblings during childbirth.

Generally, Johnston (1980) suggests that these practices can be accepted by the nurse until a consensus decision is reached with the parents as to continuance or modification. These four categories provide the nurse with a useful, cognitive means of evaluating different styles of culturally based health behaviour. In reality, however, few practices can be evaluated as absolutely fitting into one category or another.

Transcultural Children's Nursing

Brink (1976) defined transcultural nursing 'as nursing within and across cultural contexts', as health and healing do not take place within a vacuum. Transcultural nursing is designed to help nurses incorporate cultural concepts, theories and research findings into nursing practice and into nursing education.

The child-care nurse practitioner will need to be aware and responsive to the many cultural cues given by the child and family in the day-to-day care context situation. It is impossible for the nurse to be knowledgeable about the whole spectrum of cultural diversities found in any one situation, but by being informed and sensitive to these issues the nurse will be able to provide care that is appropriate, meaningful and acceptable to the child and the family within the context of their culture. Dobson (1991) describes this as 'culturally appropriate nursing care'.

The nurse may find it helpful to use the following questions as part of the care plan assessment in eliciting the family's perceptions of the child's illness and related cultural beliefs:

- What do you think caused the problem?
- Why do you think it started when it did?
- What do you think your child's illness does to him?
- How severe is your child's illness? Will it have a short or long course?
- What kind of treatment do you think your child should receive?
- What results do you hope to receive from this treatment?
- What are the major problems your child's illness has caused for you?
- What do you fear most about your child's illness? (Brunner and Suddarth, 1991)

Finally, a knowledge of developments, psychological and sociological theories to assist in the understanding of the meaning of sickness and ill health for the child and family is necessary. But it is also important to recognise their view of health or of the sickness experience. This view will be derived from a complex network of beliefs, values and cultural factors. The child's, the young person's or the family's view may be interpreted quite differently from the biomedical-orientated health-care worker's perspective or view of the same episode.

References

Ahmet, L. (1990) 'A model for midwives: support for ethnic breast feeding mothers', *Midwives Chronicle and Nursing Notes*, January: 5–7.

Barn, R. (1990) 'Black children in local authority care: admission patterns', *New Community*, 16(2): 229–46.

Bohay, I. Z. (1991) 'Cultural care meanings and experiences of pregnancy and childbirth of Ukrainians', in M. Leininger (ed.) *Culture Care, Diversity and Universality: a Theory of Nursing*, New York: National League for Nursing Press.

Brink, P. J. (1976) *Transcultural Nursing: a Book of Readings*, London: Prentice-Hall.

Brunner, L. S. and Suddarth, E. (1991) (adapted by B. Weller) *The Lippincott Manual of Paediatric Nursing*, 3rd edn, London: Harper Collins.

Cameron, E., Badger, F. and Evers, H. (1988) 'Old, needy and black', *Nursing Times*, 84(32): 38–40.

Davitz, L. L. and Davitz, J. L. (1985) 'Culture and nurses' inferences of suffering', in L. A. Copp (ed.) *Perspectives in Pain*, Edinburgh: Churchill Livingstone.

Dobson, S. (1991) *Transcultural Nursing*, London: Scutari.

Eisenbruch, M. (1988) 'The mental health of refugee children and their cultural development', *International Migration Review*, 22(2): 282–300.

Helman, C. G. (1990) *Culture, Health and Illness*, 2nd edn, London: Wright.

Johnson, M. R. D. (1986) 'Citizenship, social work and ethnic minorities', in S. Etherington (ed.) *Social Work and Citizenship*, Birmingham: British Association of Social Workers.

Johnston, M. (1980) 'Cultural variations in professional and parenting patterns', *Journal of Obstetric, Gynecologic and Neonatal Nursing*, 9(1): 9–13.

Kareem, J. and Littlewood, R. (1992) *Intercultural Therapy*, Oxford: Blackwell Scientific Publications.

Kleinman, A. (1980) *Patients and Healers in the Context of Culture*, Berkeley: University of California Press.

Leininger, M. (1981) 'Transcultural nursing: its progress and future', *Nursing and Health Care*, 11(7): 365–71.

Linton, R. (1940) 'Acculturation', in R. Linton (ed.) *Acculturation in Seven American Indian Tribes*, Gloucester, MA: Peter Smith.

Mares, P., Henley, A. and Baxter, C. (1985) *Health Care in Multiracial Britain*, London: Health Education Council/National Extension College.

Niederhauser, V. (1989) 'Health care of immigrant children: incorporating culture into practice', *Paediatric Nursing*, 15(6): 569–74.

Office of Population Censuses and Surveys (OPCS) (1990) *Population Trends*, London: HMSO.

Payer, L. (1990) *Medicine and Culture*, London: Victor Gollancz.

Thiederman, S. (1986) 'Ethnocentrism: a barrier to effective health care', *Nursing Practice*, 11(8): 52–4.

Williams, C. and Jelliffe, D. (1972) *Mother and Child Health: Delivering the Services*, London: Oxford University Press.

Zola, I. (1973) 'Pathways to the doctor – from person to patient', *Social Science and Medicine*, 7: 667–89.

COMMUNICATION IN THE HEALTH CARE OF CHILDREN

Terry Phillips
University of East Anglia

The Relationship between Speakers' Expectations and Their Ability to Make Sense, p. 108 – The Effect of Ethnicity, Gender and Class on Communicative Potential, p. 109 – Communication in a Health-care Context, p. 114 – Making the Change to a 'Communicative' Context, p. 117 – References, p. 119

The Relationship between Speakers' Expectations and Their Ability to Make Sense

The extent to which we are able to make sense of what is being said and done in a conversation depends upon our expectations about its possibilities. Conversation is both a complex social activity and an intensely personal one. As individuals we communicate to exchange information, to make sense of the world for ourselves, and to reach some form of common understanding with the people to whom we talk. But when we engage in conversation we are also part of a group, and so are involved in a social process which has 'rules' which we cannot ignore. We know these rules, not because they have been spelt out for us, but because we have become familiar with them through our general experience of conversation in a wide variety of situations. The rules have become habituated into our conversational practice – part of what Bourdieu calls our 'habitus' (Bourdieu, 1977). It follows that the wider the range of experiences we have had as speakers, the greater our potential for extracting maximum meaning from any given communication event. It also follows that speakers with limited or particular experience may encounter difficulties in conversation with people whose expectations are different because of their wider perspective.

Conversational practices are never acquired in the abstract, but developed through real interactions in concrete situations. By encountering situations of the same type over and over again we come to recognise the typical patterns of interaction which adhere to particular sorts of event. Where we cannot recognise a

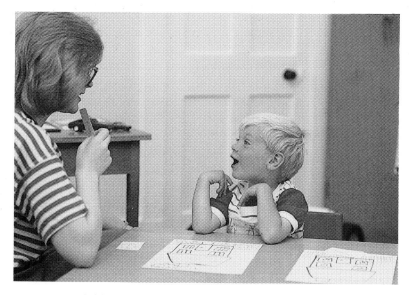

Figure 7.1   Children develop conversational skills through real interactions

situation type, we find it difficult to make sense of what is being said. Anyone invited to a formal ceremony for the first time, for instance, will have little idea about how to address people, of what might give offence, or what might be heard as appropriate. Similarly, a person who has never been in hospital before will be unable to predict the sorts of things the doctors and nurses are likely to say and will have only a slight notion of how they themselves should respond. In both cases, the newcomer's limited knowledge of the genre (the accepted pattern of interaction and the 'normal' conversational rules) makes it almost impossible for them to engage in the interaction in the same way as someone who is a 'regular'. The outcome is that they either finish up tongue-tied or they make a stab at coping with the new demands they face and risk committing blunders and appearing to be ignorant. The potential for effective communication increases in proportion to the extent that speakers share knowledge of the genre within which their current conversation event belongs.

The Effect of Ethnicity, Gender and Class on Communicative Potential

To be a good communicator a speaker must have what Hymes calls 'communicative competence' (Hymes, 1972). This term describes a speaker's *potential* for communicating effectively. Unlike performance, which is a one-off, situation-specific activity, competence must be demonstrated across a wide range of social, interpersonal and cultural contexts. The ability to recognise and respond appropriately to different genre is a part of that competence. Of equal importance is the ability to identify and accommodate to the particular conversational practices of different social groups. Every one of us belongs to a number of subcultural groups, and our conversational expectations are highly influenced, for instance, by whether we are male or female, black or white, affluent or poor, a manager or an operative, a professional or a technician, and by whether we belong to a group who come together to pursue an interest, work or education. From inside any of these groups we see the world slightly differently from anyone outside them and develop different expectations about the possibility of conversation. What counts as 'normal' communication behaviour in one subculture may be perceived as aberrant by those in another. Crossing from one subculture to another can render a speaker temporarily incompetent.

Women talking with other women will expect to do things in their conversation which men talking together will not. Nurse teachers will have slightly different conversational expectations from nurse practitioners. Male nurse teachers will probably have markedly different conversational expectancies from female nurse practitioners. People's expectations about what they are able to do with their language, and their perceptions of the value of conversation as a means of getting their point across, are not only constructed through interaction, but constructed differently according to the groups to which they belong. And in turn, the world of the group itself is shaped through conversation. The communal world, in that sense, is a 'construct' brought into being through talk itself (Halliday, 1978; Ricouer, 1984).

The social practices of one ethnic group may differ from those of another, and therefore the socially constructed conversational norms may differ too. The way a child responds when an adult speaks to them will depend in part upon the normal practice of the ethnic group from which the child comes. A child from a white Caucasian culture will keep a slight physical distance from the person with whom they are holding a conversation and will certainly not put their faces next to the other person's. An Arab child, on the other hand, will naturally approach to within a few inches of the person they are addressing in a way which to the Caucasian feels like an invasion of personal space. Children from some Asian cultures will be ashamed to look an adult in the eye or initiate a conversation because it is considered impertinent in their society. In an Anglo-Saxon culture an averted gaze denotes guilt, and unwillingness to take part in a conversation signals sullenness. An adult who did not know the cultural norms and practices of the child could make unfounded assumptions about the child.

While conversational practices engendered by ethnicity are peculiar to particular communities, those which are created by gender differences cross boundaries. Girls from a wide variety of ethnic backgrounds are socialised into expecting to respond to turns in conversations with males rather than to initiate them, and certain words and topics are conventionally prohibited from their conversation. Their contributions to a conversation are often characterised by an end-of-utterance rising intonation pattern which, because of its similarity to the tone used to ask questions, suggests tentativeness. They are often indirect when expressing concern or dissatisfaction, continuing to be polite and remain conciliatory by using modalities (such as 'perhaps', 'possibly', 'maybe') and modal auxiliary verbs (like 'might', 'could', 'may') to soften the strength of their complaint. And they avoid talking about certain topics because 'those are not the sorts of things girls talk about' (Tannen, 1986). In many cultures, linguistic habits such as these have become accepted as characteristically female. The smaller number of girls who have grown up in a community or family with an alternative set of conversational conventions to these will be perceived as acting in a masculine way. The consequence is that any girl who is direct, habitually initiates turns, introduces prohibited terms, or regularly uses a sharply falling intonation at the end of a contribution, will often be heard as intending to be aggressive.

As with gender, so with class. The conversational expectations of boys and girls who come from close, traditional families or who live in areas where many people share the same experiences and have a strong allegiance to common values, will take for granted that others within their network will understand what they have to say without the need for elaboration (Bernstein, 1971). They will give narrative accounts, the most common forms of which are found in gossip, more often than expositional ones, stories being a natural way of sharing experience and comparing values without having to fill in all the background details. For gossip, although often thought of pejoratively as something malicious, is merely a prototypical form of story-telling which allows the exploration of feelings and values. For traditional communities, stories and anecdotes provide the most common vehicle for coming to terms with difficult experiences – for example, stories about death, family rows and major disappointments (Harding, 1937; Phillips, 1971). Each time a speaker shares a personal story with others, they reshape it slightly until eventually the painful or embarrassing event which it is about becomes manageable. The young child's story begins to centre on the attention they received when they twisted their ankle instead of the searing pain that preoccupied them at the time. Anecdotes and stories are extremely versatile, however, and as well as providing a focus for the exploration of emotions they are also an important medium for making sense of new information. It is possible to explore, even savour, new 'facts' by incorporating them in stories (Rosen, 1984). The fact that close communities tell anecdotes and share stories often, means that the children in those communities *expect* to order their world through narrative accounts rather than expositional ones in which the cause of everything that happens is made explicit using the language of consequence, cause and effect, and so on (Phillips, 1991).

Traditional communities prefer narrative to discursive accounts because for them the former create solidarity and the latter suggest distance. When speakers move outside their communities to talk with professionals they often find the way these people speak creates a social distance. The young child who is used to explaining how they got a cough by telling a story – 'Me and Carol played out yesterday ... it was freezing ... even when we'd been back for half an hour ... and we were up in my bedroom drawing patterns in the steam on the window ... I could only just feel my fingers' – is liable to feel alienated by the health-care professional who uses a non-narrative mode, even though in doing so they may not include any difficult or technical language: 'According to your mother the reason why you have this cough is that you have been neglecting to wear your vest, although in my opinion it's because of the poor ventilation in your bedroom which gives rise to condensation, with the consequence that an unhealthy atmosphere has developed there.'

Unfortunately, the imperative for clear, concise information-giving amongst those who belong to the health-care culture is so strong that any child who attempts to tell a story about their experience is liable to be heard as 'holding up the main proceedings', and any nurse who encourages it for more than a brief moment will be seen as inefficient.

All social groups have their own cultural practices, and establish their own 'rules'. Over time members of a group learn the appropriate non-verbal behaviour (gesture, facial expression, gaze, posture), proxemics (physical nearness), and paralinguistics (tone, loudness) for conversation between members of the group. They also learn what may be talked about and what is proscribed. These practices affect communication because communication is itself a social practice. Our society is culturally diverse, with a range of cultural practices and a consequent variety of communication 'norms'. The linguistic diversity and difference in our society is a natural feature which offers evidence of cultural evolution. In any process of change there are opportunities for misunderstanding. When speakers brought up in one linguistic community try to interpret the actions of a speaker from another community, they are likely to gloss the other person's conversational behaviour from their own cultural-centric position. This can lead to *mis*interpretation. Our own practices are so much second nature to us that it is difficult not to try to make sense of what other people do and say in terms of our deeply ingrained conversational expectations.

Communication, then, is not a simple business of message transmission for which there is a universal set of do's and don't's that can be applied across all contexts. It is a complex social activity in which interpretation plays a major part. Not only do speakers have to interpret and make sense of each other's words, gestures and intonation, but also to understand the communication event itself. They have

- to recognise the genre in which they are operating,
- to identify the conversational practices of the subcultural group whose natural genre it is, and
- to determine how it relates to their own sub-group practices.

To communicate effectively carers must be able to avoid construing behaviour which is a consequence of inexperience in health-care settings – such as a child's apparent unwillingness to respond to questions, and their readiness to offer unasked-for personal information – as uncommunicative or disruptive. Professional competence includes the ability to communicate with children in ways that recognise and draw upon the experience they do have rather than the ability to press them to conform in situations with which they are entirely unfamiliar. The development of that competence is assisted by a knowledge of the way children use language across a range of contexts, and of how they vary it to meet the demands of particular situations, purposes and relationships.

Communication in a Health-care Context

So far we have explored some of the things which can affect the potential to make meaning and to understand speakers across a range of contexts. Now we must consider some of the additional factors which impinge on the communicative competence of children, particularly when they are communicating with health-care professionals in health-care environments.

As most children come across doctors and nurses somewhat irregularly, they are obliged to guess at how they will behave, but they do have models on which to draw. Those models are the people who have specialist knowledge, and also the authority to 'set rules'. Through their interactions with these people children have developed an understanding of the material and social worlds, and have also learned how the status of information is linked to the status of the person providing it. Some children learn, for instance, that information can be built up through joint enquiry, others that it is something which others have and will pass on to them when ready. Some learn that there are reasons for rules and that events have an explicable causal base. Others find that rules are there 'because someone more powerful than me says so', and that the happenings of the world are apparently irrationally or personally motivated. One set of children will *expect* to ask questions, the other group will often not see any point in doing so. It is clear that through their earliest interactions children are socialised into different expectations about talking with adults (Bernstein, 1971).

All children, whatever their experience of adult–child interaction, are more actively engaged when talking in their homes than in other institutional contexts. In their homes they often initiate conversations using questions, and the conversations are most often about real and immediate tasks. Like all conversationalists they face difficulties from time to time in gaining attention and in completing a turn, but they are able to experiment with strategies for handling such problems. Recordings of 2- and 3- and 4-year-olds in conversation with their parents show quite clearly that they systematically try out a range of conversational ploys to achieve an end (MacLure and French, 1981; Wells, 1981). All children, therefore, demonstrate the potential to be *actively* engaged in the process of reaching better understanding through conversation, although some children have less opportunity for doing so than others.

When children enter school at around 5 they learn to become 'pupils'. They are taught how to take part in classroom conversations, a process which involves a quite different set of competences from those they have developed spontaneously and incidentally in their earliest years. In most instances, within one term of being in school they learn not to initiate exchanges, to respond in an appropriate manner when nominated, and to expect to be *taught* information rather than build it through mutual exploration. They learn, too, that teachers ask closed questions to which the answer is already known (MacLure and French, 1981). The longer a child is in school, the greater their socialisation into the school culture, and into the highly stylised turn-taking pattern that encourages receptiveness rather than activeness (Barnes, 1976; Sinclair and Coulthard, 1975). Much of the interaction in the classroom context becomes ritualised, and communication becomes as much about correct performance of those routines as about in-creasing understanding. If children regularly experience inter-actions with an adult as occasions for receiving information from an 'authority' – that is, someone who 'knows' – they may develop into 'expert' listeners, but they are rather less likely to feel able to offer their own information without first being given permission.

Some adults, of course, do offer children the opportunity to ask questions about the information presented to them. They are often disappointed that their invitation is not taken up. It is not surprising, however, that a child who has come to see in-formation exchange as a process of transmission and reception in which adults are the transmitters and children the receivers, does not suddenly become an enthusiastic interrogator of the 'taken-for-granted' who is critical of the discourse they hear around them (Phillips, 1984) – that is, someone who asks questions about either the substantive context or the status of the information being offered. As far as the child is concerned, information from an adult is axiomatic; because an adult has said it, it is like that. The child will see nothing unusual about adults asking them questions to check the validity of their account, but would not expect to question the adult's. There is no apparent function for *interrogating* questions from them in conversation with adults who have both knowledge and authority.

Despite an increasing degree of care for children in the community, much child health care – like schooling – continues to take place in an institutional context. And even where it does not, the relationship between adult caregiver and young recipient is still largely one of authority figure to subordinate. Just as in school, children become less competent than at home because they perceive the conversational 'rules' as different from those they use with their family and peers, so they become unable to realise their full communicative potential in hospital, surgery or clinic because of the way in which the conversational practices there are significantly unlike those through which they have accumulated and absorbed their repertoire of expectations. If health-care professionals are to promote an expectation among children who present for medical attention that they will be able to talk about their care in a way which will lead to understanding of what is to happen to them, a key task will be to encourage them to 'deconstruct' the situation in which they find themselves. In other words, the professional's focus will need to be on the situation in the first instant, and on the information only after it has been demonstrated convincingly to the child that the current situation is different from other apparently similar ones.

For carers working in hospitals, the major call will be for presentation of information in a way that encourages children to express their feelings and anxieties and offers them an opportunity to make sense of it in relation to their previous experience. For those working in the community, or in local practices, or in some other kind of primary health-care team, the focus might be more on health promotion and education than on information about what has been discovered and decided about the child's illness. However, all health-care professionals who work with children are, whether they like it or not, in the business of education. Health and wellness are promoted through increased understanding, on the one hand, and the development of a culture of interest in healthy life style, on the other. A visit to a health-care professional, whether for treatment for a chronic condition, acute surgery or something more minor, is a learning opportunity. That learning can be either well-informed or ill-informed, depending on the extent to which the child is able to explore information about the world, themselves and health. The opportunity for such exploration does not depend on good information transmission alone, but upon the creation of a context in which information is naturally explored, personal responses welcomed, and matters of interest to the child placed high on the agenda. This context cannot happen out of nowhere or in an instant. Unless a child has been encouraged during her conversation with adults to say how what she has been told makes her feel, she is unlikely to reveal her worries. Similarly, if her whole experience of talking with adults is one in which what she is told is axiomatic, she is unlikely to either challenge the validity of what has been proposed, or – less strongly – to explore it. What is taken for granted by an expert adult may not be at all obvious to a child who may find the information difficult to understand, startling, unbelievable, curious, fascinating or even interesting enough to want to find out more.

Making the Change to a 'Communicative' Context

It is clear from what has been said about the need for a climate of exploration and enquiry that improved adult–child communication in health-care settings is dependent on changes in the conversational context more than upon the development of technical speaking and listening skills. Communication is affected by the fact that the health-care professional has authority by virtue of being an adult – which affects *the interpersonal tenor* of the conversation (Gregory and Carroll, 1978); by the fact that the child is also in a client/patient role – which affects *the functional tenor* (Gregory and Carroll, 1978); and by the asymmetry of experience which each participant brings to the health-care setting. These three factors mean that the child has much less opportunity for exploiting the communication potential of the genre than the adult, an imbalance of opportunity which cannot be redressed merely by the adult getting better at what *they* do. Because communication is interactive, if the child does not perceive the new opportunities offered to them, there will be no improvement in the communication.

What, then, must health-care professionals do to improve their communication with children and ensure that they become active participants in the promotion of their own health and well-being? As demonstrated earlier, they must at the very least change their conversational practices in ways that recognise what the children bring to the conversation. But although essential, this is not sufficient to guarantee better communication. When a child has built up expectations over many years these will not simply go away because an adult has chosen on a single occasion to do something different. The innovation will be interpreted as if it were an aberrant form of the old practice unless the wider conversational opportunities offered by the new circumstances are explicitly revealed to the child. If we want children to understand through their communication, health-care professionals must first help them to *decon*struct the communication event they find themselves in, and then work with them to *re*construct it as an occasion for collaborative meaning making.

In practical terms, deconstruction requires the adult to set out clearly at the beginning of the conversation what the new ground rules are and show how these differ from the ones the child might have expected. The statement of new ground-rules will not wipe out in one afternoon what a child has learned over time, of course, but provided the contrast with habituated practice is made clear, the possibility for something different will have been opened up. If a child is told,

> I will stop from time to time to ask you if you have any questions, and when I do I will wait a few seconds so that you can have time to think. Normally children don't query what nurses tell them, but I hope you will because I really want to hear what your concerns are,

they will know that they can legitimately interrogate what otherwise would have to be taken for granted. If they are told,

> Sometimes I shall ask you to tell me the story of how you did something. Nurses often don't have time to listen to stories but today I'm just going to sit back and listen while you tell me everything you can remember about it,

they will know that they can appropriately use narrative. In each case, the explicit contrast with previous 'norms' begins the process of deconstruction through which the child is not just invited to change their conversational practice but actually given some idea of how to do it. Reconstruction, on the other hand, will be accomplished through the conversational practice itself. Adults can help children take a full part in health-care-related conversation by intervening as little as possible themselves and using back-channel noise ('uh-huh', 'mmm', and so on) and prompts (like 'go on', 'would you like to say a little more about that?') to encourage them to talk. And they can, of course, introduce anecdotes of their own to initiate the anecdotal mode. Perhaps most usefully of all, they can invite the child to co-construct an account of the child's condition in which details are included from the child's perspective whether or not the nurse thinks them irrelevant.

References

Barnes, D. (1976) *From Communication to Curriculum*, Harmondsworth: Penguin.

Bernstein, B. (1971) *Class, Codes, and Control*, London: Routledge and Kegan Paul.

Bourdieu, P. (1977) *Outline of a Theory of Practice*, Cambridge: Cambridge University Press.

Cazdan, C., John, V. and Hymes, D. (eds) (1972) *Functions of Language in the Classroom*, New York: Teachers' College Press.

Gregory, M. and Carroll, S. (1978) *Language and Situation*, London: Routledge and Kegan Paul.

Halliday, M. (1978) *Language as Social Semiotic: the Social Interpretation of Language and Meaning*, London: Edward Arnold.

Harding, D. (1937) 'The role of the onlooker', in *Scrutiny*, 6(3): 247–58.

Hymes, D. (1972) Introduction in C. Cazdan, V. John and D. Hymes (eds) *Functions of Language in the Classroom*, New York: Teachers' College Press.

Kearney, R. (ed.) (1984) *Dialogues with Contemporary Continental Thinkers: the Phenomenological Heritage*, Manchester: Manchester University Press.

MacLure, M. and French, P. (1981) 'A comparison of talk at home and at school', in G. Wells (ed.) *Learning through Interaction*, London: Cambridge University Press.

Phillips, T. (1971) 'Poetry in the junior school', in *English in Education*, 5(3).

Phillips, T. (1991) 'Creating contexts for exploratory talk', in D. Wray (ed.) *Talking and Listening*, London: Scholastic.

Phillips, T. (1984) 'Exploratory talk: a critical learning discourse' in P. Scrimshaw (ed.) *Spoken Language and New Technology*.

Ricouer, P. (1984) 'The creativity of language' in R. Kearney (ed.) *Dialogues with Contemporary Continental Thinkers: the Phenomenological Heritage*, Manchester: Manchester University Press.

Rosen, H. (1984) *Stories and Meanings*, Sheffield: NATE.

Sinclair, J. and Coulthard, M. (1975) *Towards an Analysis of Discourse: the English Used by Teachers and Pupils*, London: Oxford University Press.

Tannen, D. (1986) *That's Not What I Meant: How Conversational Style Makes or Breaks Your Relations with Others*, London: Dent.

Wells, G. (1981) 'Becoming a communicator', in G. Wells (ed.) *Learning through Interaction*, London: Cambridge University Press.

Wray, D. (1991) *Talking and Listening*, London: Scholastic.

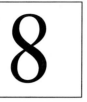

8

HOSPITALISATION AND DEVELOPMENT

Bruce Lindsay
Norfolk College of Nursing and Midwifery
and
Helen Meehan
Queen Elizabeth Hospital, King's Lynn

Hospitalisation is seen increasingly as a 'last resort' strategy in the health care of children (Department of Health, 1991). The problems which even a short period of hospitalisation can create for children and their families are well recognised (Affonso *et al.*, 1992; Easterbrooks, 1989). Alternative strategies, such as day procedure units and community children's nursing services, are slowly becoming established, with their benefits being recognised by individual carers and by organizations. In this chapter discussion will focus on the possible effects of hospitalisation on the development of one particular group: infants, especially those requiring admission to neonatal units (NNUs) immediately after birth or in the first few weeks of life. Within this chapter the term 'infant', meaning 'a child in the first year of life' (Department of Health, 1993) is the one most commonly used to refer to the children who are nursed on neonatal units. This is because a significant percentage of NNU patients remain on such units beyond the neonatal period (the first twenty-eight days of life) and continue to be affected by this environment.

Despite the move towards the community care of sick children, over 90 per cent of children in Britain are delivered in hospital and spend the first hours or days of their lives as 'in-patients', despite being well. Those needing special or intensive care enter a world even further removed from the home environment. Infants admitted to hospital after days or weeks at home must adapt, along with their families, to fresh surroundings and routines. The care they receive may well be life-saving, but its effects on the development of the infant and family may be detrimental to the quality of that life.

We will consider the possible effects of hospitalisation on infant development in some detail. We will go on to ask what those who work with hospitalised infants and their families can do to maximise the benefits of admission and minimise any potentially detrimental effects. Can an acute hospital stay have benefits for a infant's development beyond the treatment of a physiological problem? Or is the most we can hope for a 'holding operation' which attempts to prevent regression or delay and minimise post-discharge problems for the infant and family?

The Developing Child: Expectations and Needs

Children are expected to develop. Caregivers, older siblings and health professionals all have expectations for this development. Such expectations may be based on previous child-rearing experiences, on information from caregivers and friends, or on a knowledge of developmental research and personal study.

Whatever the expectations for an individual child's development, the child is unlikely to meet them exactly. The child's uniqueness, the environment in which development takes place and the combination of influences upon that development combine to ensure that, as yet, there is no sure way of predicting development. However, research findings do allow us to identify age ranges during which the majority of children will achieve certain observable 'milestones'.

Authors subdivide development in a number of ways. Bee (1989), for example, discusses the development of 'the physical child', 'the thinking child' and 'the social child'. Taking a more holistic, if less scientific, approach it can be said that our expectations for development can be summarised in three words: more, better and new.

More is expected of a child in terms of growth: more height or weight, more steps while walking, more words in the vocabulary, more independence in feeding or dressing. We also expect a child to become better, or more skilful, for example in co-ordinating movements, in speaking or in remembering songs. New skills and activities are also expected in the developing child. Indeed, in the early months something new may be expected by the parents almost daily. Once the child demonstrates a new skill we go on to expect more of it and at a higher standard.

In some instances we expect less, of course: fewer primitive reflexes, less sleep, less crying. But this is usually secondary to the new or increased abilities or behaviours we expect as a result: new voluntary activities, more wakefulness or better communication.

Although we expect children to develop, we do not expect them to do so spontaneously. Children need warmth, nutrition and good hygiene to survive and grow. Development requires even more from the environment.

The developing infant needs stimulation. The physical world should contain sights, sounds, tastes, smells, shapes and textures to stimulate the senses, to encourage movement and exploration, to reward new skills. The social world needs other human beings to enable communication and interaction, to develop early skills of transmitting and interpreting information, to encourage the developing personality and cognitive skills.

The infant also needs an environment where interactions with caregivers can develop. Attachment and bonding must take place, not only for the good of the child but also for the parents and other family members. The environment must be one which allows, if not enables, such relationships so that normal development can continue in the years to come. Physical closeness, during feeding, bathing or play, 'conversations' with the carer, an understanding of the infant's behaviours on the part of the parents (and vice versa): all these are seen as vital aspects of development in this early period of life.

Early development, then, can be said to be at least in part a product of the environment in which it occurs. Desirable environmental factors would, therefore, be those which positively encourage development to take place: adequate food, warmth and cleanliness; a small number of primary carers, able to quickly learn to understand the infant; interesting things to see, hear, taste or touch; physical and psychological safety, without smothering any desire for exploration and adventure. Good health and financial security for all members of the family complete the ideal. A social network offering the infant the chance to interact with people from outside the immediate family and giving the caregivers opportunities to seek support or advice from trusted and experienced others will enhance family development.

An infant who requires hospitalisation, particularly during the neonatal period, throws the plans for a secure, cosy, nurturing home environment into chaos. Whether the health problem is short- or long-term, acute or chronic, life-threatening or merely 'inconvenient', it disrupts expectations and threatens the environment. A hospitalised infant pressurises the family socially, financially, psychologically. Life in the specialist unit is an alien one. Multiple carers, barriers to physical contact, necessary changes to routines of feeding, sleeping or bathing all serve as obstructions to the creation of a developmentally desirable environment. Or so the current beliefs of health carers seem to suggest. But what effects does hospitalisation have on early development? How detrimental, or desirable, is a stay in hospital for the infant? Have we now recognised and acted to remove the major problems associated with hospital admission or are the more insidious effects still largely unacknowledged?

Early Development: a Contemporary Image

Most babies born in contemporary Britain are born in hospital. The Peel Report (Ministry of Health, 1970) recommended that facilities be made available for 100 per cent of births to take place in hospital. The shift from home deliveries was so effective that by the early 1980s less than 1 per cent of births were carried out at home. While this figure is now on the increase, birth is now rarely an event experienced within the family's home and shared by the local community: it is instead an activity which takes place within specialist units, controlled to a greater or lesser extent by health-care professionals for whom each baby is one of hundreds or even thousands who begin their lives in the unit each year.

The stereotyped, romanticised image of the early months seems little affected by the move from home to hospital birth. The happily married parents return to their comfortable, well-prepared home to care for the baby. The family, including older siblings, grandparents and others, take responsibility for the twenty-four hour care of the new arrival who develops well within this optimal physical, social and psychological environment. Regular health-care interventions ensure that the baby is well protected from childhood diseases, while the stimulation of the surroundings results in the early achievement of developmental milestones.

Of course, this idealised image of early life is neither universal nor necessarily the best for the baby. Babies live, grow and develop successfully in an almost infinite number of settings, and it is probably a rare child whose life is spent in an unchanging family setting. Indeed, the possible home circumstances in which a baby may grow up are so diverse that no accurate prediction of their effect on the baby's development or of optimal circumstances is possible. As a result, an accurate assessment of

the effect which a period of hospitalisation in the first weeks of
life will have on development is even harder to achieve.

'Normal development'

An understanding of normal development is essential if we are
to consider the implications of hospitalisation for that development. But what is 'normal development'? One thing must be
clearly understood: normal development is not about absolute,
fixed measures but about observable ranges of behaviours,
achievements or physical measurements. In other words, the
normal 1-year-old is not x cm tall and y kg in weight, but has a
height and weight which both fall within an acceptable range of
measures. The normal child does not walk at exactly x months
of age but at some point within a range of ages.

What is considered normal, it should also be remembered, is
neither universal nor unchanging. Normal physical parameters
vary between countries, while any detailed assessment of the
physical development of an individual infant should take into
account the physical characteristics of that individual's biological parents. Acceptable physical development also varies
with time, for example, the normal range of birth weights in late
twentieth-century Britain differs from that to be found in the
early years of the eighteenth century. Other elements of development have seen accepted definitions of normality over-
turned in recent years. Neonatal sensory abilities, physical
co-ordination and communication skills have been seriously
underestimated until recently, when the advent of modern
audio-visual equipment has enabled researchers to study these
abilities more closely. Far from being a *'tabula rasa'*, or 'clean
slate', the infant is now recognised as an active participant in life
from birth, with skills and abilities previously believed to appear at a much later stage.

To complicate matters further authorities are far from
unanimous about development and the factors which influence
it. 'Normal development' is not clear-cut, and the effects which
various environments may exert on it remain open to question.
So how can we as carers of infants make any worthwhile assessment of the effects of hospitalisation? A starting point may well
be the identification of ways in which the hospital environment
changes the interactions between the infant and the 'outside
world'. Following this we can go on to identify which aspects of
development may be affected by these changes and to what extent this may result in long-term alterations to these aspects.

The effects of hospitalisation _____

For many babies, life outside the mother's womb begins with medical intervention. All babies are assessed immediately after birth, and the midwife or doctor's first comments about them may remain with the parents for years to come. When a paediatrician or other assistant has been called to attend a delivery because it is thought that the baby will need assistance, the baby may well be placed upside down on the resuscitation equipment before the need for any intervention has been established. Unnecessarily vigorous resuscitative measures may cause problems and result in more medical interventions being required. Tew (1990) looks at the results of the British births survey of 1970, and notes the fact that breathing problems were more often suffered by and more often proved fatal to babies born in hospital, even though a much greater proportion of them were transferred to neonatal units. This would seem to suggest that, as soon as the moment of birth, hospitalisation has an effect on potential development.

Most babies need no active intervention to help them cope with their changing environment. As the baby is delivered, the first examination is occurring to confirm that this is so. The midwife visually scans the baby looking at colour, muscle tone, response and effort to breathe. A gentle hand on the baby's chest will feel the heartbeat. The information obtained by this assessment will often be used and documented formally as the Apgar Score (see Figure 8.1) which represents the condition of the baby at one and five minutes. After a short while, ideally in the presence of the parents, the midwife carries out a systematic physical examination to confirm normality or promptly to refer for paediatric assessment.

In the hours and days following birth each baby undergoes further assessment by midwives and doctors to confirm as far as possible that all is well. The mother is involved too, reporting the passage of urine and meconium, the first stool and feeding patterns. A mother may be the first person to notice if the baby is not behaving in the way that she expects, but her care may well be guided by the professionals around her and inhibit her from the more natural interaction that she may experience at home. Most babies make the transition to life outside the womb successfully, and go home within the first few hours or days of life. On transfer home the community midwife and general practitioner will care for mother and baby, and at between ten and twenty-eight days, as their

Sign*	Score		
	0	1	2
Heart rate	Absent	Slow (below 100)	Fast (above 100)
Respiratory effort	Absent	Slow Irregular	Good Crying
Muscle tone	Limp	Some flexion of extremities	Active
Reflex irritability (stimulation of foot or oropharynx)	No response	Grimace	Cry, cough
Colour	Blue Pale	Body pink Extremities blue	Completely pink

*The first two, heart rate and respiratory effort, are the most important.

Figure 8.1   The Apgar Score

needs change, the health visitor replaces the community midwife. Over the following months contact with health-care professionals diminishes and the parents usually become gradually more independent from the health-care system.

We still know little about the effects of hospitalisation on the development of babies born in hospital, or its effects on the early child–parent relationship. In the years following the Peel Report there has been a downward trend in perinatal mortality and morbidity, but it is difficult to assess the degree to which the move to hospital births has been responsible for this. Tew (1990) in her *Critical History of Maternity Care* discusses this fully. Many other factors seem to influence outcome; for example, social class or uptake of antenatal care. How much of the improvement is due to the immediate availability of expert medical care for babies born compromised is open to question. We do know that some routine practices introduced in an attempt to increase the likelihood of a safe delivery may actually cause complications rather than avert them. Continuous foetal monitoring is still carried out routinely in many maternity units, but there is no research which shows that it has contributed to the decline in perinatal morbidity. Although the incidence of cerebral palsy has not decreased (Stanley and Blair, 1991), the incidence of instrumental or operative intervention has greatly increased, bringing more attendant risks of iatrogenic problems. Soft tissue injury, lacerations and bruising may be associated with Caesarean section or instrumental delivery (O'Doherty and Avery, 1985). Anaesthesia or analgesia administered to the mother may affect the baby's ability to breathe. Fractures, organ damage or nerve injuries may occur due to twisting or stretching at delivery. Foetal scalp electrodes have been known to cause trauma to babies' heads, misplaced cord clamps can cause soft tissue injury. Oxytocic drugs have been known to be administered to infants in error with disastrous consequences. In some cases problems caused by these interventions may lead to admission to a NNU.

Hospitals are not healthy places. Babies have immuno-globulin G (IgG) transferred to them via the placenta in the last trimester of pregnancy, but they have little resistance to common organisms such as staphylococci or streptococci, which can be found on the skin and in the throats and noses of those caring for them. Midwives and doctors moving between mothers and babies may carry pathogenic organisms. Air and dust in hospitals may harbour bacteria resistant to commonly used antibiotics. Soiled sanitary pads and nappies may encourage bacteria to breed. The infant's eyes and cord stumps are very vulnerable to infection, while intact skin offers the best barrier to invading organisms. Any breaks in the skin caused perhaps by birth injury need to be observed for signs of infection and treated swiftly: hospital-acquired infections may prove life-threatening. An awareness of the potential dangers of the hospital environment is essential to practitioners so that they can identify problem areas and work to minimise the problems and maximise the benefits of the hospital environment.

Future physical development of the infant will be dependent on the nutrition that is supplied. There can be little doubt that the best food for human babies is human milk. Although the majority of women in Great Britain today choose to breast-feed (64 per cent in the Infant Feeding 1985 OPCS Social Survey Division), many abandon breast-feeding in the first two weeks. Midwives are available during this time to support and promote breast-feeding, yet by four months only 26 per cent are still fully breast-feeding (DHSS, 1988). Such an opportunity to make a positive contribution to the future health and development of each baby requires further exploitation.

In the Neonatal Unit

The main focus of our discussion will be the time spent in a neonatal unit. While such admissions are necessary to help infants to overcome early problems which may threaten life, the neonatal unit is a unique and frightening world for the baby and caregivers alike. Its possible effects, over and above its role in overcoming the infant's physical problems, may remain with the child and family for life.

Infants admitted to NNUs have a problem or problems needing skilled health-care interventions. At a time when the majority of babies are enjoying the beginnings of their relationships with their families at home, or when others are still some weeks away from delivery, the infant in the NNU must cope not only with the physiological problems which necessitated admission but also with the unit's own unique and inhibiting environment.

The technology and care activities needed to enable these infants to survive lead in themselves to the creation of what is probably one of the least recognisable and most threatening of hospital settings for the relatives: a 'chaotic and highly technical' setting (Affleck *et al.*, 1989), which is as far removed from the norm for an infant as one can imagine, and one which is even more awesome for the new mother still recovering from the stresses of childbirth.

The primary aim of the neonatal unit is to enable the infant to survive and go home as well and as quickly as possible. In achieving this aim the damage done to the infant's development and to the development of relationships between the infant and other family members could be irreversible. But in basing its care on more than just enabling the infant to survive, the contemporary NNU may well offer an experience to the family which has positive benefits.

The physical environment of an NNU offers a wide range of barriers to normal development. Incubators provide life-saving protection for the infant but also create an isolated living space. Sounds from outside, particularly human voices, are distorted by the incubator shell and must appear very strange to the infant's ears. In turn, the infant's cries are muffled and distorted to those outside: recognising and differentiating those cries is thus harder for the caregivers. In an exploration of how the NNU sounds to a preterm infant, Thomas (1989) explores how intense sounds can directly damage the cochlea permanently. The incidence of sensorineural hearing impairment is 4 per cent in low birth-weight infants and 13 per cent in very low birth-weight (VLBW) infants. The incidence among all infants is 2 per cent. The lighting, temperature and humidity within the incubator are controlled within tight limits, denying the infant the

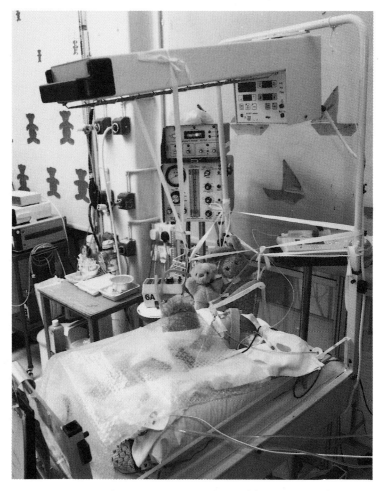

Figure 8.2 'Hi-tech' care in a neonatal unit: life-saving care brings its own problems for normal interaction

chance to live within a normal pattern of light and dark, heat and cold, moist and dry (Mann *et al.*, 1986).

While in the NNU the infant may find that much of the time is spent receiving uncomfortable or even painful treatments or procedures. Time for cuddles, play or feeding may of necessity be minimal. During periods of high dependency the infant may be attended to by many different people over the course of the day, with time spent with mother or father being only a small percentage of the total time.

The unit creates problems for the families too. The lack of time which they can spend in normal interactions with their new baby is likely to conflict with their expectations of their first weeks together. The fact that for much of this time they may be able only to see or touch, rather than cuddle or play with the baby will serve to increase this conflict. When the infant needs skilled care from the unit staff the parents may experience feelings of alienation and uselessness, adding to the problems already existing for their attempts at bonding. Beneditti *et al.* (1977) suggest that the machinery in the NNU may be seen by the mother as a source of rivalry: a new uterus more able than she to nurture the baby. This leads in turn to a desire for the machinery to fail, creating guilt feelings in the mother as a result.

The infant may well suffer further restrictions as a result of treatment. Infusions, monitors, endotracheal tubes and probes will limit freedom of movement and the ability to cry. Normal oral feeding may be impossible, preventing normal sucking. Eyes may be covered to protect the baby from ultra-violet light, restricting early visual development and creating yet another barrier to the establishment of social relationships.

The intimidating environment, aversive procedures and intrusive monitoring result, according to Levy-Shiff *et al.* (1989), in the emotional withdrawal of parents and in estrangement from the infant. This problem is heightened by the mother's loss of self-esteem which results from the production of a non-healthy baby (Jeffcoat *et al.*, 1979). During the time on the NNU the parents may well develop reluctance to participate in care and may show dependence on unit staff (Cagan, 1988), becoming defensive and reluctant to visit.

The NNU environment, created to ensure the continued existence of individuals who would otherwise be incapable of life, may also put the early development of these infants at risk. An NNU which aims solely at the treatment of the infant's physical problems may well achieve a high degree of success at this: in recent years this success has been so great that the gestational age of viability has been lowered from twenty-eight to twenty-four weeks. But a truly effective NNU also seeks to optimise its possible effects on the early development of its patients and their carers.

Maximising the benefits of the NNU is a twofold process: first, ensuring that the possible adverse effects are minimised, and secondly making the best possible use of the facilities and staff available. To minimise adverse effects they must first be identified. This is a difficult process, for the adverse effects of the NNU must be differentiated from the effects of low birth weight, prematurity or pathology.

Preterm infants have an increased likelihood of neurological damage, mental retardation or cerebral palsy and may develop difficulties with language, visual perception, visual-motor integration, short attention span and hyperactivity even when intelligence is normal (Avery and Glass, 1989). VLBW infants may also display retarded psychomotor or cognitive development, although recent studies show a decreasing percentage of VLBW infants with these problems (Bollea, 1986). VLBW infants do not interact with their carers as well as term infants of normal weight, and this can put a strain on relationships within the family. Bernard *et al.* (1984) found that mothers of VLBW infants initially spent longer with them in the early months following discharge. However, by the end of the first year interactions were lower than those with normal, term infants: they suggest that this was because of poor reinforcement of the mother's behaviours by the infants. An earlier longitudinal study (Blake *et al.*, 1975) found that mothers of the VLBW infants studied were anxious and over-protective. The infants, 160 of whom took part in the study, were themselves more likely than average to be timid, hyperdependent and anxious. Over the longer term the VLBW child has been identified as continuing to display problems. Minde *et al.* (1989), for example, note that 'intellectually normal very small premature infants ... are frequently reported to have moderate behavioural problems ... at 48 months'.

The NNU as a 'Caring Environment'

For the well baby the home environment is clearly seen as the best place to be. Mills *et al.* (1988) state clearly that the evidence supporting this notion 'is hard to refute'. Improving the NNU as a caring environment is likely therefore to be achieved at least in part by increasing its resemblance to the home environment, while preserving its ability to provide high-quality health care.

Making the physical appearance of the NNU more 'user-friendly' may be one useful strategy. Within the stark setting of the incubator the infant can be stimulated and comforted by the presence of soft toys of various materials and textures, by the use of patterned linen and sheepskin pads, or by the placing of photographs or pictures on the incubator cover within the infant's line of sight (Stewart, 1991). Allowing the infant to suck a dummy may also be beneficial, speeding up the development of a sucking reflex, enhancing weight gain and helping the achievement of mouth feeding, all of which ultimately reduce the length of stay in the NNU (Bernbaum *et al.*, 1982).

The NNU itself can be made to appear less clinical by careful use of decor, lighting, choice of curtain materials. A unit which encourages the infant's relatives or carers to visit and take part in care will help to maintain their self-esteem by ensuring that they remain aware that they have a valuable role to play while the infant stays on the NNU (Hunsberger, 1989). An atmosphere which ensures that information can be freely exchanged will also help to promote a partnership in the baby's care and treatment and will make best use of information gained from observation of the infant.

Two aspects of NNU care appear crucial for the development of the infant and the new relationships between the infant and family: interactions between the family and the NNU team, and the interactions between the infant and the carers (whether they are unit staff or family members). Modern medical and nursing care means that the vast majority of infants admitted to NNUs are eventually discharged home. As the parents will eventually assume responsibility for the care of their child it is in the best interests of future family confidence and security that they are involved and supported in the provision of care as soon as they feel able. Indeed, Levy-Schiff *et al.* (1989) emphasise that the parents are crucial in the successful development of the premature infant, providing a vital element in caregiving, 'social enrichment and encouragement'. But they also note that the hospital nursery which they studied offered few opportunities for parent–infant social interaction.

There would seem to be a need for staff and parents to foster an interdependence in promoting the psychological and emotional well-being of families. McHaffie (1990) stresses the importance of staff seeing events as parents see them, and discusses the importance of recognising the individual perspectives each visitor will have of what is happening. She also calls for combining technological skills with a real understanding of psychological needs, combining care of the infant with care of the family and for an expansion of community follow-up care. There is also some evidence to suggest that parental responses to the baby's admission to the NNU may differ in fathers and mothers. Hock *et al.* (1989) believe that separation anxiety 'is experienced differently in fathers and mothers'. They view maternal separation anxiety as a 'personality disposition' heightened or lowered by the reasons for the separation and by infant characteristics (for instance, whether the infant is sick or well). The baby in the NNU is likely to be a major source of separation anxiety.

In a detailed study of infants in an Israeli preterm nursery (a unit which did not give intensive, high-technology care but acted instead as a 'transitional care unit'), Levy-Schiff *et al.* (1989) found marked differences between the mother– and father–infant relationships. The infants were preterm but not small for dates and had no serious medical problems or deformities. All had arrived early, before the parents were psychologically or practically ready for their arrival. The study found that, overall, mothers visited more often and for longer than fathers (no information about residential status of the parents was given). This result in itself is unlikely to cause anyone surprise, but the roles of the parents during visiting were of interest. Initially, mothers took part in markedly more caregiving, talking and holding than did the fathers. However, by discharge the disparity between the parents was virtually nil. Mothers continued to give the majority of the care, but fathers were recorded as taking the lead in playing with and stimulating the infant. These later contacts, according to the researchers, 'paralleled those of parents of full-term infants'.

Encouraging parents to participate in care demands of the NNU staff the ability to recognise those aspects of care which can become part of the parents' role. But it also demands of these staff the confidence to develop parents' skills in areas which would normally be considered the domain of the qualified health professional. This is particularly vital in cases where the baby will need ongoing care following discharge – for example, of a tracheostomy or oxygen therapy. Even where this is not the case, involvement in specialist care may well help to increase parental confidence and self-esteem and to assist parent–infant relationships to develop.

One of the first roles of the caregivers to be challenged when the infant is admitted to the NNU is that of feeding. Throughout pregnancy the feeding of the newborn baby will have been an important topic, with antenatal care probably placing great emphasis on promoting breast-feeding. In some cases breast-feeding may already have started before the baby's admission to the NNU. Wherever possible, the continued promotion of breast-feeding should be part of the unit philosophy. Where the infant is unable to suckle, the mother can be supported in expressing her breast milk as a supplementary feed to establish and maintain lactation (Stine, 1990).

Increasingly, evidence is being produced to support the idea that the way in which the infant is dealt with on the NNU has a bearing on the eventual success of treatment and care. Some interventions will profoundly affect future development. Photo-therapy poses potential risk of retinal damage (Moseley and Fielder, 1988). Watson (1991) discusses how scarring caused by thoughtless placement of chest drains and sticking plaster may disfigure and result in severe breast distortion in adulthood. Turrill (1992) discusses how important good positioning of pre-term infants is, to help prevent skeletal and motor deformities.

Positioning of infants will often be dictated by their health problems. In many cases this may mean that infants lie prone, despite the fact that this runs counter to current advice regarding safe positioning of infants, which suggests that they should lie on their backs or sides (Department of Health, 1993). The Chief Medical Officer's Expert Group does recognise that some infants – for example, those at risk of airway obstruction or those with breathing difficulties – should be nursed prone (Department of Health, 1993), and the monitoring and observation available in the NNU allows this to be done safely. However, parents must be clearly informed of the reasons for the nursing of their baby in the prone position and must clearly understand whether or not this should continue after discharge home.

While the most effective approach to care will, of course, vary from infant to infant, some general principles do appear to be applicable. High levels of light, noise or touch appear to upset the sick or preterm infant, while infants as young as ten days show a response to a change in caregivers (Hunsberger, 1989). Gentle rocking or touching seems to be beneficial, however, with gentle stroking or massage reducing the incidence of apnoea and bradycardia as well as increasing auditory response (Helders *et al.*, 1988). Schaefer *et al.* (1980) suggest that early stimulation may enhance psychomotor development in the pre-term infant.

Short-term considerations

Contemporary nursing theory views our patients or clients as 'whole people', to be cared for as individuals rather than as collections of health problems. Contemporary child-care nurses, taking this belief one stage further to encompass whole families, undertake care with the intention of meeting a wide range of needs, beyond physical care alone. For the infant on the NNU this means that the time spent as an in-patient is time during which the pain and discomfort of the illness and treatment are minimised as far as possible by skilled nursing care of the whole family. Such care should go beyond the minimalisation of problems and should help to begin the sound relationship between the parents and the infant which de Chateau (1980) views as vital for the effective use of this early period of life. In contrast to the care described by authors such as Robertson and Robertson (1989), infants in NNUs today should find that their feelings of pain, discomfort and insecurity are recognised and that their needs for communication, safety and comfort are identified and met.

Long-term problems

However effective care in the NNU may be at bringing about a successful resolution to the infant's physical problems and at minimising the adverse effects of the treatment and care, there is evidence that longer-term problems persist in the months and years following discharge when mothers may experience painful memories of hospitalisation (Affleck *et al.*, 1989). It is also possible that the extensive 'professional' care experienced by the infant may lead to later patterns of attachment similar to those found by Belsky and Rovine (1988). Their study, of normal children receiving care from babysitters or day centres, found that these patterns of attachment 'are commonly regarded as evidence of insecurity'.

Long-term recovery

Other research emphasises the resilience of the young child and suggests that long-term problems following discharge from the NNU are less of a problem than at first thought. Easterbrooks (1989), for example, states that despite interactional problems caused by factors such as hospitalisation the preterm infant is able to form secure attachments to the mother and is as likely as a term infant to form such an attachment to the father. This finding is supported by the work of Minde *et al.* (1989), who found the distribution of attachment patterns in VLBW infants at 12 months of age to be very similar to that of term infants. Sluckin *et al.* (1983) also support this view. They conclude that following a stay in a NNU 'there is no evidence that the mother's feelings towards her infant are in any way permanently distorted'.

Greenberg and Crnic (1988) found that by a corrected age of

2 years VLBW infants who were otherwise healthy had caught up with term, normal weight infants in all except motor skills. Rutter (1989), in a detailed review of factors affecting early development, suggests that the effect of early adversities (such as hospitalisation) is less than might be expected because very young infants have yet to develop strong attachments. They are thus protected from the worst of the effects of separation. Rutter emphasises strongly the influence of the infant's subsequent life experiences: 'Even markedly adverse experiences in infancy carry few risks for later development if the subsequent rearing environment is a good one.'

Further support for this more optimistic view of development comes from Bradley (1989). He criticises much of the research into child development undertaken in the previous thirty years, particularly that carried out in the laboratory, 'the social equivalent of a desert island'. His criticisms include theories of mother–infant bonding, which he describes as 'a myth' which fits neatly into accepted male ideas of child-rearing as women's work. For Bradley, research which seeks to show that early traumas have predictable effects for later life generally fails to do so. The concept of later problems stemming from inadequate bonding and attachment is not, he claims, supported unless the poor bonding and attachment are followed by consistently poor home environments. Bradley, like Rutter, believes that even early trauma due to prematurity or severe neonatal illness will have very different developmental outcomes according to the home circumstances.

Contemporary evidence appears to support the notion of children as resilient beings, able to bounce back from early setbacks to catch up with their more fortunate fellows in most areas of development before entering school. So the long-term effects of early hospitalisation seem not to be as adverse as they may at first appear.

But does this mean that approaches to care in NNUs need not be as carefully thought out as was at first suggested? Of course not. One thing to remember about much of the research cited in this chapter is that it took place in NNUs, or with children who had been treated in NNUs, which aim to do far more than just solve the physical problems of the baby. In other words, modern research uses modern neonatal units and is thus influenced by the success of their approaches to care.

If we return to past practices, dealing solely with the infant's physical problems, excluding the family from involvement in care and doing nothing to meet the developmental, psychological or social needs of the infant, and then repeat this research, we may well find far less evidence for successful developmental progress following discharge.

There are, clearly, enough possible problems to be overcome during the period of stay on the NNU to make a carefully considered approach to care of vital importance. The stresses placed upon the infant and family as a result of the infant's health status or of the treatment necessary for a successful outcome are enormous. Any NNU should work towards their minimisation: such an approach is the right of the infant and of the family. As health-care professionals we have a responsibility to ensure that we are aware of our potential for enhancing the development of each child we care for and limiting the negative effects that hospitalisation may have. A great deal of research over the past twenty years has changed the way that we view, for example, the bonding process and much research continues into the physical, social and emotional experience of the infant. Those caring for infants should nurture their own knowledge so that their provision of care and professional growth reflects the same healthy development as they aim to promote.

References

Affleck, G., Tennen, H., Rowe, J., Roscher, B. and Walker, L. (1989) 'Effects of formal support on mothers' adaptation to the hospital-to-home transition of high-risk infants: the benefits and costs of helping', *Child Development*, 60: 488.

Affonso, D. D., Hurst, I., Mayberry, L. J., Haller, L., Yost, K. and Lynch, M. E. (1992) 'Stressors reported by mothers of hospitalized premature infants', *Neonatal Network*, 11(6): 63.

Avery, G. B. and Glass, P., (1989) 'The gentle nursery: developmental intervention in the NICU', *Journal of Perinatology*, 9(2): 204; cited in MIDIRS *Midwifery Digest* (1991), 1: 3.

Bee, H. (1989). *The Developing Child*, 5th edn, New York: Harper and Row.

Belsky, J. and Rovine, M. J. (1988) 'Nonmaternal care in the first year of life and the security of infant–parent attachment', *Child Development* 59: 157.

Beneditti, P., Mayer, R. and Galletti, F. (1977) 'Il problema psicologico del monitoraggio e del follow-up del bambini "nati a riscio"' *Neuropsichiatria infantile*, 192–3: 921–49; cited in Kaminski *et al. Perinatal Care Delivery Systems: Description and Evaluation in European Community Countries*, Oxford: Oxford University Press, 1986.

Bernard, K. E., Bee, H. L. and Hammond, M. (1984). 'Developmental changes in maternal interaction with term and pre-term infants', *Infant Behaviour and Development* 7: 101.

Bernbaum, J., Pereira, G. and Peckham, G. (1982) 'Increased oxygenation with non-nutritive sucking during gavage feeding in premature infants', *Paediatric Research*, 16, 278A Abs. 1199.

Blake, A., Stewart, A. and Turcan, D. (1975) 'Parents of babies of very low birth weight: long term follow-up', in R. Porter and M. A. O'Connor (eds) *Parent–infant Interaction*, Amsterdam:Elsevier.

Bollea, G. (1986). 'Review of evaluative studies of intensive care for very low birthweight infants – psychological aspects', in Kaminski, M. *et al. Perinatal Care Delivery Systems; Description and Evaluation in European Community Countries*, Oxford: Oxford University Press, 1986.

Bradley, B. S. (1989) *Visions of Infancy: a Critical Introduction to Child Psychology*, Cambridge: Polity Press.

Cagan, J. (1988) 'Weaning parents from intensive care unit care', *American Journal of Maternal Child Nursing*, 13 (4): 275–7.

De Chateau P. (1980) 'Parent–neonate interaction and its long-term effects', in E. C. Simmel (ed.) *Early Experiences and Early Behavior*, New York: Academic Press.

Department of Health (1991) *The Welfare of Children and Young Persons in Hospital*, London: HMSO.

Department of Health (1993) *The Sleeping Position of Infants and Cot Death*, London: HMSO.

Department of Health and Social Security (1988) *Report on Health and Social Subjects, No. 32, Present day Practice in Infant Feeding*, London: HMSO.

Easterbrooks, M. A. (1989) 'Quality of attachment to mother and to father: effects of perinatal risk status', *Child Development*, 60: 825.

Greenberg, M. T. and Crnic, K. A. (1988) 'Longitudinal predictors of developmental status and social interaction in premature and full-term infants at age two', *Child Development*, 59: 554.

Helders, P. J. M., Cats, B. P., Van der Net, J. J. *et al.* (1988). 'The effects of a tactile stimulation/range finding programme on the development of very low birth weight infants during initial hospitalisation', *Child Care, Health and Development*, 14(5): 341.

Hock, E. McBride, S. and Gnezda, M. T. (1989) 'Maternal separation anxiety: mother–infant separation from the maternal perspective', *Child Development*, 60: 793.

Hunsberger, M. M. (1989) 'Nursing care during hospitalization', in R. L. R. Foster., M. M. Hunsberger, and J. J. T. Anderson (eds) *Family-centred Nursing Care of Children*, Philadelphia: W. B. Saunders.

Jeffcoat, J. A., Humphrey, M. E. and Lloyd, J. K. (1979) 'Disturbance in parent–child relationship following pre-term delivery', *Developmental Medicine and Child Neurology*, 21: 344.

Klaus, M. H. and Kennell, J. H. (1982) *Parent–infant Bonding*, St Louis: C. V. Mosby Co.

Levy-Shiff, R., Sharir, H. and Mogiliner, M. B. (1989) 'Mother- and father preterm infant relationship in the hospital preterm nursery', *Child Development*, 60: 93.

Lewis, M. and Volkmar, F. (1990) *Clinical Aspects of Child and Adolescent Development*, Philadelphia: Lea and Febiger.

McHaffie, H. (1990) 'Their child–our patient', *Paediatric Nursing*, 2(8): 23.

Mann, N. P., Haddow, R., Stokes, L., Goodley, S. and Rutter, N. (1986). 'Effect of night and day on preterm infants in a new born nursery: randomised trial', *British Medical Journal*, 293(6557): 1265.

Mills, B. C., Matlock, J. R. and Herrell, A. L. (1988) 'Infant care – does anybody care?' *International Journal of Early Childhood*, 20: 36.

Minde, K., Goldberg, S. Perrotta, M. *et al.* (1989) 'Continuities and discontinuities in the development of very small premature infants to 4 years of age', *Journal of Child Psychology and Psychiatry and Allied Disciplines*, 30: 391.

Ministry of Health (1970) *Domiciliary Midwifery and Maternity Bed Needs: The Report of the Standing Maternity and Midwifery Advisory Committee, Sub-committee Chairman, J. Peel*, London: HMSO.

Moseley, M. J. and Fielder, A. R. (1988) 'Phototherapy: an ocular hazard revisited', *Archives of Disease in Childhood*, 63: 886.

O'Doherty, N. and Avery, M. E. (1985) *Atlas of the Newborn*, 2nd edn, Lancaster: MTP Press.

Robertson, J. and Robertson, J. (1989) *Separation and the Very Young*, London: Free Association Books.

Rutter, M. (1989) 'Pathways from childhood to adult life', *Journal of Child Psychology and Psychiatry and Allied Disciplines*, 30: 23.

Schaefer, M., Hatcher, R. P. and Barglow, P. D. (1980) 'Prematurity and infant stimulation: a review of research', *Child Psychiatry and Human Development*, 10(4): 199.

Sluckin, W., Herbert, M. and Sluckin, A. (1983) *Maternal Bonding*, Oxford: Basil Blackwell.

Stanley, F. J. and Blair, E. (1991) 'Why have we failed to reduce the frequency of cerebral palsy?' *Medical Journal of Australia*, 154(11): 623.

Stewart, A. J. (1991) 'Mums and dads need care too: supporting parents of babies in neonatal units', In Glasper, A. (ed) *Child Care: Some Nursing Perspectives*, London: Wolfe.

Stine, M. J. (1990) 'Breastfeeding the newborn: a protocol without bottles', *Journal of Human Lactation*, 6(4): 167.

Tew, M. (1990) *Safer Childbirth? a Critical History of Maternity Care*, London: Chapman and Hall.

Thomas, K. A. (1989) 'How the NICU environment sounds to a preterm infant', *American Journal of Maternal/Child Nursing*, 14(4): 249.

Turrill, S. (1992) 'Supported positioning in intensive care', *Paediatric Nursing*, 4(4): 24.

Watson, S. (1991) 'What would you do? Baby friendly care on NNUs', *MIDIRS Midwifery Digest*, 1(4): 479.

PART 3

MOVING FORWARD

9

NURSING: CONCEPTS, THEORIES AND MODELS

Stephen Happs
Anglia Polytechnic University

Background

Historically nursing was subservient to medicine, and the content of nursing courses was often based on medical specialities. As a result of adhering to this 'biomedical model' patients (including children) were perceived as physical beings, with little attention being paid to their wider needs. The effect of this lack of attention on children is well documented by writers such as Robertson and Robertson (1989), while Pearson and Vaughan (1986) identify four outcomes of using this model:

1 Routinisation – policy and procedure books in which prescribed routines are laid down;
2 Physical care – a concentration on the physical aspects of care – technical skills are ascribed a greater status than other skills such as communicating or comforting;
3 Because little attention is paid to providing for individual needs, then 'getting through the work' is often the primary objective of nursing teams;
4 Care versus cure – cure is the major objective of the biomedical model, and this also then becomes a goal for nurses who subscribe to this approach. However, it has significant implications for those who work in areas where curative outcomes are not possible.

Adam (1983) identifies a major problem emerging from this allegiance to medicine: 'For nursing to justify its claim to being an independent health profession offering a particular service to society, it must adopt its own conceptual base.' This chapter considers nursing's adoption of such a conceptual base, surveying the nursing literature to explore the interrelationships between concepts, theories and models from a broad perspective to help in an understanding of their specific application to the nursing care of children.

Nursing: Art or Science?

Meissener (1981) suggests that the sciences seek to answer 'how' questions, whilst in contrast the arts attempt to find answers to 'why' questions. For nursing, this contrast has produced a perennial debate: nursing – art or science?

The view of nursing as a science is a fairly recent development. The arguments supporting nursing as a science or as the applications of science have gathered momentum. This has had the effect of reducing the view of nursing as an art. Interestingly, nursing degree courses are more commonly found to be Bachelor of Science rather than Bachelor of Art. Although there has been an appropriate emphasis on research as a means for extending nursing knowledge, Crowe (1981) notes that, whereas the technicalities of research may be specifically scientific, the recognition of the problem and the questions to be asked are an art dependent upon the imagination of the researcher. Nursing as an art form has elements in common with other art forms (dance, music, painting and sculpture) (Peplau, 1988). Its aim is to produce favourable changes within patients through nursing actions. Pagana (1987) has described nursing as the 'conscience of the health care system'. This lends support to the notion of advocacy, nurses functioning as the keepers of the morality and ethics of patient care. Curtin (1979) echoes this view by asserting that nursing is a moral art. The American Nurses Association (ANA, 1980) supported the view of nursing as a science by declaring that an occupation becomes a profession when its practitioners use scientific knowledge to understand and to treat the phenomena within its socially delegated domain of service.

Stainton (1982) states that 'Science seeks to understand the real world. Theory is the product of science: research is its tool.' Science has an important part to play in nursing; indeed Riehl and Roy (1974) advocate that 'effective nursing action depends upon predictions that are based on scientific principles'. They oppose alternative approaches suggesting that 'Unfortunately many of our actions are still based on intuition'. In contrast to this view, Merrabeau (1992) asserts that 'The nursing profession has tended to devalue particularistic, craft-based knowledge in favour of the more generalisable, discipline-based knowledge'. The basic theories of nursing which constitute the normal science of the nursing profession are in the form of facts and theories. Such knowledge names and describes a particular phenomenon. Nursing, including child-care nursing, can therefore be viewed as a science or an art, or perhaps more appropriately as a combination of both.

The debate over nursing as science or art will no doubt continue. However, it is my view that the two are inseparable. The most effective nursing can only be achieved if both the art and the science of nursing are retained, fully developed and incorporated into nursing practice.

Nursing Process

Nurses are moving away from a medical model to a more systematic method of planning and delivering individualised care. This is referred to as the nursing process and has been defined as 'a deliberate intellectual activity whereby the practice of nursing is approached in an orderly, systematic manner' (Stanton *et al.*, 1985). The nursing process therefore provides order and direction to nursing care. There is general agreement amongst authors that there are four phases, or components, necessary for the nursing process: assessment, planning, implementation and evaluation. However, the nursing process is not a panacea for all nursing problems. There are difficulties inherent in it; this has been exacerbated in Britain by its hasty and, in many cases, clumsy introduction. McFarlane (1986), commenting on the introduction of the nursing process and models, states: 'They landed the practitioners in the nursing process predicament, and now the models muddle.'

A key point and one which needs emphasising, as it is pivotal in understanding the thrust of nursing models, is this: the nursing process and models of nursing are not the same thing. They are related to each other but their purpose is different. Aggleton and Chalmers (1985) assert that the

> Nursing process needs to be informed by a particular understanding of the needs of patients and how best these may be met. Without this, the nursing process might unwittingly be used to plan and deliver care around medical concerns and not those relating more specifically to nursing practice.

Clark and Bishop (1988) provide a useful analogy, and suggest that models of nursing and the nursing process can be likened to the body and engine of a car: 'The nursing model provides the structure or framework for nursing care. The nursing process is the driving force. A car without an engine is a useless frame, but given an engine it becomes an effective machine.'

Often nurses appear to conduct an assessment without any agreed guiding framework. It is accepted that all of us have a private image of nursing (Reilly, 1975). However, as Reilly goes on to say, 'In turn, this private image influences our interpretations of data, our decisions, and our actions.' Little wonder that when moving from assessment through to planning difficulties begin to emerge. It seems to me that the assessment phase has become a creative writer's dream. No longer are we satisfied with 'Fractured femur due to road traffic accident'; rather, we resort to 'Compromised musculoskeletal system occasioned through vehicular trauma'. However, both miss the key point – these are not specifically nursing problems.

Much energy has been wasted on writing complex care plans that fail to identify the key area for nursing. Of course, this is not to suggest a universal picture nor one which denigrates any particular individuals; rather, it is a reflection of the problems inherent in trying to plan care without a framework. Many nurses are left feeling impotent and vulnerable. Because they have no conceptual model to base care on, the assessment is off course, therefore the plan is difficult to devise. This leaves the practitioner wondering what they are supposed to be doing apart from the obvious high-visibility tasks and/or caretaking duties. In the environment of child-care nursing it can also leave the family wondering what is supposed to be done and, perhaps more crucially, *why* things are being done. A sensible, constructive evaluation is almost impossible to carry out as there are a myriad interpretations. This is not to suggest that the nursing process is in any way a defective tool; rather, that without a guiding framework it is, to borrow an analogy, an engine with nowhere to go.

Concepts, Theories and Models

Many practitioners seem to find the whole issue of models and theories a somewhat sterile academic exercise. Gould (1989) sums it up thus:

'Nursing is, after all, a practice discipline, and it seems indefensible that new ideas should be thrust upon those at the sharp end, responsible for direct patient care, by academics or managers who, though genuinely concerned by these issues, do not face the everyday realities associated with implementation.

McFarlane (1986) also notes that the ideas come from those who no longer are involved in the practice of direct patient care. This has meant that 'those who practise nursing for real are left to incorporate these new ideas into their practice with little help'.

This view is reinforced by some of the complex terms used by predominantly North American theorists, yet if nursing models serve no other purpose than to lend support to particular academics then they are in my opinion worth very little. However, if the purpose of these models is to aid nurses in providing a framework for their care, then indeed there must be some point in considering them. Akinsanya (1984) makes the point that the link between theory and practice is not an academic exercise. It is essential to the sustenance of a theory-based, knowledge-dependent practice. In a later text (Akinsanya, 1989), he offers advice to those coming to this area for the first time: 'The truth is that every science has its own particular terms, concepts and principles which are essential for the development of its knowledge base.' Many nurses understand the language of the medical model because they are so familiar with it. The need to come to terms with a new language, that of a nursing model, can be seen as yet another barrier to the development of this base.

Some texts make little distinction between concepts, theories and models. Whereas this may, at first impression, make it easier to understand, it may well cause confusion later on. Therefore they will be considered separately.

Concepts

Concepts are variously defined but a general picture does emerge. Harre (1966) suggests that concepts are vehicles of thought that involve images. Chinn and Jacobs (1983) define concepts as 'a complex mental formulation of an object, property or event that is derived from individual perception and experience'. Torres and Yura (1974) state that concepts are a symbol or general notion whose function is to generally classify objects, events and processes. Toffler (1974) suggests that impressions received by sensing our environment evolve into concepts. Concepts can occur on a continuum from the more directly experienced (empiric) through to the abstract. In order to make this more clear, imagine you have admitted a child to hospital. An example of empiric concept could be the child's eye colour; it is directly observable. The blood pressure of that child is not directly observable but remains relatively empiric as standardised instruments are available. However, if one were to grapple with the notion of the child's 'wellness', this would lead into much more abstract concepts. These highly abstract concepts are sometimes referred to as 'constructs' (in that they are constructed from many sources of direct and indirect evidence).

Theory

Again, many writers have chosen to define theory in different ways. However, consideration of these should lead to a greater understanding of the term 'theory'. The word evolves from the Greek word *'theoria'* which is similar to a 'vision'. Torres (1985) suggests that 'the development of theories should be viewed as rational and intellectual and leading to the disclosure of truth'. This involves comparing, experimenting and the uncovering of relationships, and gives rise to a systematic view of a phenomenon that is explanatory and predictive in nature. If true predictability is achieved, theories become laws (for example, the law of gravity).

Stevens (1984) states that a theory 'is a statement that purports to account for or characterise some phenomenon'. Childcare nursing theory should try to explain or describe the phenomenon called 'child-care nursing'.

Theories therefore are different from concepts: theories are made up of concepts but are tested so that 'one can separate the critical and necessary factors (or relationships) from the accidental and unessential factors (or relationships)' (Stevens, 1984).

Models

Models are not the real thing, but they attempt to represent the reality of it. Models are not only confined to children's toys; many models are created in professional lives. Nor are they only confined to tangible things: many organisations use 'computer models' in order to perceive some future reality. Therefore models of nursing are 'a descriptive picture of practice which adequately represents the real thing' (Pearson and Vaughan, 1986). There is a distinction to be made here between a conceptual model and a theoretical model. Fawcett (1978) views a conceptual model as a compilation of highly abstract, related concepts. A theoretical model deals with concepts that are narrower in boundary and scope and derive from research. For this chapter the terms 'practice model', 'nursing model' and 'models of nursing' relate to conceptual models, defined as sets of concepts and the propositions that integrate them into a meaningful configuration. This makes them highly abstract and general and not 'limited to any specific individual, group, situation, or event' (Fawcett, 1989). Popper (1959) cautions against generalities; if something is too general it is of little use. The statement 'Your child will grow taller' tells you virtually nothing. However, the statement 'Your child will grow to a height of 1 m 75 cm' is of much more use. However, one should not assume that models are therefore without use. They act as a guiding framework, not a highly prescriptive tool.

What, then, is the relationship between conceptual models and theory? Aggleton and Chalmers (1985) state that nursing models lack the strength to be called theories of nursing. However, as Adam (1983) points out, 'a conceptual model specifies nursing's focus of inquiry and may thus lead to the development of theories which will prove useful not only to nurses but to other health professionals as well'.

Due to the abstract nature of conceptual models, many theories are required to describe, explain and predict. In a similar way many conceptual models are required to explain the discipline of nursing.

Disciplines single out certain things which they deal with in a unique way. This is the most global perspective and is even more abstract and general than a conceptual model. This is termed the 'metaparadigm' of the discipline (Kuhn, 1977). Therefore each discipline's metaparadigm is the first level of distinction between them. However, it is not unusual for more than one discipline to be interested in similar concepts.

The Metaparadigm of Nursing

The central concepts of the discipline of nursing are person, health, environment and nursing (Torres and Yura, 1974). Fawcet (1989) notes that the metaparadigm of nursing has been 'evolving since Nightingale ... first wrote of nurses' actions in relation to environmental influence on the person's health'. Some writers have extended the notion of four metaparadigm concepts. However, these works 'underscore the centrality of person, environment, health and nursing (as activity or action)' (Fawcett, 1989).

World-views _____

Before considering each of the metaparadigm concepts in more detail, a mention of world-views seems appropriate. World-view refers to some of the underlying beliefs about the nature of the relationship between person and environment found in a conceptual model. Two sets of opposing world-views will be covered: the mechanistic and organismic.

These two views are logically incompatible; a mechanistic world-view suggests passivity and reactivity, whereas an organismic world-view speaks of activity, integration and wholeness. The mechanistic world-view supports the view of the person as a machine. They are inherently at rest and respond in a reactive way to external forces. This view is described as reductionist, and proposes that the whole is the sum of its discrete parts. Behaviour is seen as objective and therefore predictable. Changes in the person are seen as quantitative, which suggests adding or subtracting a number of parts.

In stark contrast, the organismic world-view sees the person as inherently spontaneous: a source of acts. The person actively engages in interactions, as opposed to only reacting to external forces. Cause and effect are therefore ruled out, prediction becoming tenuous. This view supports the notion of holism which puts forward the view that the living organism is an integrated, organised entity not reducible to discrete parts.

Modern approaches to child-care nursing would support an organismic world-view: the child as active and interactive. Past practices seem more supportive of a mechanistic world-view, in which children are reacting to outside forces rather than shaping them by their own activity.

Person _____

The view that nurses hold about the concept of person will have a profound effect upon their nursing actions. Sarter (1988) suggests that nursing is concerned with some fundamental questions about the nature of human beings. Thibodeau (1983) asserts that 'Defining human nature is more than a mere descriptive exercise, because human nature directly influences the natures of nursing'.

For example, nurses on a ward may ascribe different importance to a particular section of an admission form for a child: 'Has your child been baptised?' One nurse may feel it relatively unimportant that this is completed; another may feel it to be absolutely vital. This may well stem from deep-seated views of what happens following death. Neither view is 100 per cent right or wrong, but could lead to disagreement if these issues are not properly addressed.

In a book aimed to consider child care, the issue of 'person' is cast into sharp relief. If someone were to ask you, 'Is a child different from an adult?' what would your response be? On one hand a commonsense answer would be 'Of course a child is different'. They think, feel and act in ways different to adults. Indeed, they have a different status in law. However, another commonsense answer could be, 'Of course not, they are both human beings. Children become adults, they are the same – yet at different stages.' It is not the intention of this chapter to consider these responses in detail. However, Weller (1991) notes that 'Children continue to be treated as mini-adults', and goes on to state that 'This approach is emphasised by the mirroring of patterns of care based upon the adult model which deny the concept of childhood'. It is perhaps significant that there has been a marked move away from the use of the term 'paediatrics' in respect to nursing towards the notion of 'child care'. Perhaps in child care more than any other area of nursing the 'person' being cared for is not just the child. The family is actively involved and therefore the relationship between nurse and patient extends well beyond two individuals (Schultz, 1987).

Health ————————————————————————

Health has been defined in many different ways by many different authors. This chapter cannot possibly begin to review them. However, some underlying trends can be picked out. The first issue is whether wellness and illness is seen as a continuum – in other words, wellness through to illness. An alternative approach could be to perceive wellness and illness as mutually exclusive – in other words, well or ill. Again, the views individuals hold about this will affect their responses to and interactions with patients. It has been described in terms of a physical and social perspective, or in terms of behaviour. Wellness has been described in more abstract, non-behavioural terms or as a dialectical process.

Field (1972) proffers yet another view, in which a distinction is made between illness and disease. He states that illness is the person's subjective experience of ill health, whereas disease relates to a pathological abnormality. If one of the goals of nursing is to promote wellness, it is surely obvious that the definition of health used must materially affect nursing practice (Thibodeau, 1983).

Environment

Meleis (1986) considered the literature on environment and proposed this synthesised view: 'the setting, the background, and the conditions that surround and encompass the nursing client or are anticipated to do so'. In considering the conditions that surround and encompass the patient Thibodeau (1983) draws a useful distinction between the internal and external environments. Internal environment relates to such factors as 'personality, mental capacity and genetic make-up' (Thibodeau, 1983). The external environment relates to all of those forces outside the individual. Nurses are part of the human environment surrounding patients. The nature of the interactions between people and their environment also has an influence on the nature of nursing.

Nursing

As one might imagine, there are many accounts and definitions of nursing. It is clear that the view people hold about what nursing is, what actions are congruent with it, and how these should be evidenced will result in different sets of nursing behaviours. The American Nurses Association (ANA, 1980) state that 'Nursing can be said to be owned by society, in the sense that nursing's professional interest must be and must be perceived as serving the interests of the larger whole of which it is a part'. This is echoed in the UKCC Code of Professional Conduct (UKCC, 1992), which states: 'Each registered nurse, midwife and health visitor shall act, at all times, in such as manner as to: safeguard and promote the interests of individual patients and clients; serve the interests of society; justify public trust and confidence.' The ANA go on to state that nursing is 'the diagnosis and treatment of human responses to actual or potential health problems'.

Models – Benefits or Drawbacks?

As stated before, all nurses hold a picture of what nursing is, what they do and how they do it. The fact that some nurses have made their views explicit, sharing them in the wider public arena, has been 'central to the advancement of nursing as a discipline and profession' (Leininger, 1988). Fawcett (1989) asserts that 'a conceptual model facilitates communication among nurses and provides a systematic approach to nursing practice, education, administration and research'.

She also points out that there is a relationship between conceptual models and clinical practice, and asserts that 'conceptual models influence clinical practice by specifying standards ... identifying relevant legitimate recipients of nursing care ... content for the nursing process; suggesting methods for delivery of nursing services' and that 'Nursing practice in turn provides data that can be used to determine the credibility of the conceptual models' (Fawcett, 1992). A conceptual model of children's nursing, for example, informs the way in which child-care nurses approach and undertake the care of children. Practice, however, may cause the concept to be altered: perhaps from one in which the child is seen as unable to make decisions to one in which decision making by children is deemed possible. The concept is altered and in its turn goes on to influence changes in practice.

However, there are many nurses who are sceptical about the value of models. Luker (1988) has suggested that the introduction of models carries an implied criticism of current practice and that it diverts nurses' attention away from the really important issues. Many nurses to whom I have spoken see models as helping other nurses who can't quite make it on their own, 'but they're not really appropriate for me!'.

Dickoff and James (1986) highlight the fact that what is often adopted by nurses is 'a neat little digest or slogan version or sketch of the theory'. They go on to suggest that 'sometimes more time is devoted to its adoption and formal incorporation into documents of institution and curriculum than to its use' (Dickoff and James, 1986). The key to avoiding some of this is to be found in a simple yet elusive word: 'agreement'. Pearson and Vaughan state; 'Achieving agreement demands that the team as a whole consider each individual nurse's beliefs about patients and nursing work.' If this is achieved, then certain benefits will accrue:

1 consistency and continuity of care;
2 reduction in conflict within the team;
3 increased understanding by other disciplines;
4 direction for nursing care;
5 a guide in decision and policy making;

6 a guide for the criteria in selection of new team members (Pearson and Vaughan, 1986).

One model, many models or your own?

Much debate has been generated on this issue. There is a divide within the literature, some advocating a multiple model perspective, others advocating a single model approach.

In Britain there has been a strong push towards practitioners building their own models (Wright, 1990). Riehl and Roy (1980) were strong advocates of a single, unified conceptual model of nursing. However, Fawcett (1989) states that they have modified their views. An approach which endorses multiple models has certain benefits. Feldman (1980) notes that it allows 'the profession to view nursing from many perspectives, thereby increasing understanding of its nature and scope'. Another benefit is that it avoids the problem of 'premature closure on options for the discipline' (Stevens, 1984). This is also true for each individual practitioner. Kristjanson *et al.* (1987) highlighted the fact that the use of one model 'prematurely closes the perceptions of the practitioner'. Schon (1983) points out that the experienced practitioner must learn to recognise, and build up, a repertoire of ways in which situations can be framed, and methods for dealing with these situations.

Fawcett (1989) asserts that it is 'unlikely that there ever will be one unified conceptual model of nursing'. A growing idea in the area of conceptual models is the notion of theoretical pluralism. Dickoff and James (1986) warn of the dangers of moving from one model to another. This they term 'Ishmael shifts' after the character in *Moby Dick* who states, 'I must flee, sign on for another ship, going I care not where so long as it is sailing away from here'. Pluralism is not just trying out one model after another; it is acknowledging that 'there are a range of choices available in any given practice situation ... Practitioners make different choices and in so doing, select a standard against which to decide what is correct' (Kristjanson *et al.*, 1987).

Should you design your own model of nursing? This practice has gained popularity and momentum, certainly within this country. Avant and Walker (1984) encouraged practitioners to construct their own nursing models to meet specific practice requirements. MacDonald (1988), in recounting her experience, spoke of the realisation that 'We had the knowledge, commitment and enthusiasm, so we decided to create our own paediatric nursing model'.

Fawcett (189) casts doubt on Avant and Walker's advice, stating that 'There is no guarantee that new personal models would be more explicit, public or focused on nursing phenomena'. She points out that many of the published models of nursing took many years to develop. Nye and Berado (1981) suggest that several good general conceptual models 'introduce more order and are more parsimonious of everyone's time than a thousand limited, specific ones'. Fawcett (1989) goes on to suggest that nurses should continue systematically to evaluate the use of models of nursing. Their reports should be presented at conferences and in peer-review journals.

Classification of models

Various attempts have been made to classify conceptual models of nursing. Although there is no absolute agreement amongst the authors, some common features appear. The following types of models will be discussed: developmental, system and interaction.

Developmental models

Models which are described as developmental focus on the notions of growth, development and maturation. Included in these are 'theories of physical, cognitive, social, spiritual and moral development through the life span' (McFarlane, 1986). The notion of change is pivotal to developmental models. In addition to this there is also the notion of the direction of the change. A child is not an adult but a child becomes an adult through cognitive, social and physical changes. There is no absolute point at which a child suddenly becomes an adult; it is a process. As well as direction, there is also the notion of stages of development with developmental models either implicitly or explicitly indicating the force responsible for the movement along the developmental continuum.

Systems models

Systems models draw on the literature of general systems theory for explaining nursing situations. The focus of these models is the system, with consideration being given to an examination of its parts and their relationship at a particular point in time. Change in these models is of secondary importance; the key factors are the system and its environments.

A system could be a child. The parts would be made up of the organs of the body and the environment could include the family. However, the system could be the family, with the children and parents being the parts and the environment being the wider community.

The assumption of systems is that they tend to move towards a balance between internal and external forces. Systems models consider the addition or subtraction of units in relation to the target system (quantitative) as opposed to qualitative changes. Therefore actual or potential problems in the function of the system and interventions which maximise effectiveness and efficiency are emphasised.

Interaction models

These models concentrate on the nurse–patient interaction as their central theme. Symbolic interactionism is an important feature of these models as well as the notions of self-concept, role, communication and perception. McFarlane (1986) notes that 'there is a growing recognition that nurse–patient interaction is fundamental in all fields of nursing and that finding meaning in a sickness situation is something to which the nurse contributes'. Therefore identification of actual and potential problems in interpersonal relationships is the focus of these models.

A person's perception of others, their environment and surrounding events depends on the meaning attached to these phenomena. Thus perceptions are of vital importance in these models, and people communicate in order to discover each other's perceptions of particular situations.

There are other types of models identified within the literature: human needs, energy field, humanistic conservation and self-care. However, these are generally particular to one model and cannot be discussed here.

Child-care Nursing

There is, I suspect, a natural tendency to see the applicability of developmental models to child-care nursing. However, it would be folly to assume that these models should be used in these areas or that they are appropriate only for those areas. With the increasing emphasis being placed on family-centred nursing, the value of systems models becomes clear. The client may not be the child but the whole family, so models which address the family system may well have some value. Interaction models too can be seen to be applicable to child-care nursing as a great deal of discovery in terms of meaning takes place between child, nurse and family.

Some attempts have been made to consider models specifically for child-care nursing. Casey (1988) noted that there is a partnership between child, family and child-care nurse. There is an acknowledgement that, in many cases, it is the child's family who assist in meeting the needs of the child and who mediate between the child and the environment.

Barnard developed the Parent-Child Interaction Model over a number of years (see Baker *et al.*, 1989). One of the major thrusts of her work was the development of assessment tools for child health, growth and development whilst viewing the parent and child as an interactive system.

However, this should not suggest that models specifically designed for child care are necessarily superior to others. Indeed, they may be found not to fit in with a particular practice area at all well. No one model is right; no one model is wrong. At the end of the day the model chosen should serve to enhance the nursing care offered to children and their families; that is their purpose.

Finally, whatever is decided – whether to adopt a published model of nursing, an individually invented one or one generated through systematic testing – the issue of accountability is of importance. If child-care nurses are to be accountable for providing a service which they are employed to provide and for the proper use of the resources made available, then the incorporation of models into their practice must surely help to fulfil this quest. If one is to be able to account for one's actions, then they must be 'explainable, defendable and based on knowledge rather than tradition or myth' (Pearson and Vaughan, 1986). Nursing models can help towards this end. This does not mean that adopting a particular model or models will be the end to all one's troubles. However, it may mark the start of a whole new set of beginnings.

References

Adam, E. (1983) 'Frontiers of nursing in the 21st century: development of models and theories on the concept of nursing', *Journal of Advanced Nursing*, 8: 41.

Aggleton, P. and Chalmers, H. (1985) 'Models and theories: critical examination', *Nursing Times*, 81: 38.

Akinsanya, J. A. (1984) 'The uses of theories in nursing', *Nursing Times*, 80: 59.

Akinsanya, J. A. (1989) (ed.) *Recent Advances in Nursing (24): Theories and Models of Nursing*, London: Longman.

American Nurses Association (1980). *Nursing: a Social Policy Statement*, Kansas City: ANA.

Avant, K. C. and Walker, L. O. (1984) 'The practicing nurse and conceptual frameworks', *American Journal of Maternal Child Nursing*, 9: 87.

Baker, J. K., Borchers, D. A., Cochran, D. T. Kaltofen, K. G., Orcutt, N., Terry, E. G., Wesolowski, C. A. and Yeager, L. A. (1989) 'Parent–child interaction model', in Marriner-Tomey (ed.) *Nursing Theorists and Their Work*, 2nd edn, St Louis: C. V. Mosby.

Casey, A. (1988) 'A partnership with child and family', *Senior Nurse*, 8(4): 8.

Chinn, P. L. and Jacobs, M. K. (1983) *Theory and Nursing: Systematic Approach*, St Louis: C. V. Mosby.

Clark, J. and Bishop, J. (1988) 'Model-making, *Nursing Times*, 84(27): 37.

Crowe, R. (1981) 'Scientific nursing research: art and science', in J. P. Smith (ed.) *Nursing Science in Nursing Practice*, London: Butterworth.

Curtin, L. L. (1979) 'The nurse as advocate: a philosophical foundation for nursing', *Advances in Nursing Science*, 3: 1.

Dickoff, J. and James, P. (1986) 'Toward a cultivated but decisive pluralism for nursing', in M. McGee (ed.) *Theoretical Pluralism in Nursing Science*, Ottawa: University of Ottawa Press.

Fawcett, J. (1978) 'The relationship between theory and research: a double helix', *Advances in Nursing Science*, 1(1): 49.

Fawcett, J. (1989) *Analysis and Evaluation of Conceptual Models of Nursing*, 2nd edn, Philadelphia: F. A. Davis Co.

Fawcett, J. (1992) 'Conceptual models and nursing practice: the reciprocal relationship', *Journal of Advanced Nursing*, 17: 224.

Feldman, H. R. (1980) 'Nursing research in the 1980s; issues and implication.' *Advances in Nursing Science*, 3(1): 85–92.

Field, D. (1972) 'Disability as social deviance', in E. Friedson and J. Corber (eds) *Medical Men and Their Work*, Chicago: Aldine Atherton.

Gould, D. (1989) 'Teaching theories and models of nursing: implications for a common foundation programme of nurses', in J. A. Akinsanya (ed.) *Recent Advances in Nursing (24): Theories and Models of Nursing*, London: Longman.

Harre, R. (1966) 'The formal analysis of concepts', in H. Klausmerer and C. Harris (eds) *Analysis of Concept Learning*, London: Academic Press.

Kristjanson, L. J., Tamblyn, R. and Kuypers, J. A. (1987) 'A model to guide development and application of multiple nursing theories', *Journal of Advanced Nursing*, 12: 523.

Kuhn, T. S. (1977) *The Essential Tension: Selected Studies in Scientific Tradition and Change*, Chicago: University of Chicago Press.

Leininger, M. M. (1988) 'Leininger's theory of nursing: cultural care diversity and universality', *Nursing Science Quarterly*, 1(4): 152.

Luker, K. (1988) 'Do models work?' *Nursing Times*, 84(5): 27.

MacDonald, A. (1988) 'A model of children's nursing', *Nursing Times*, 84: 52.

McFarlane, J. K. (1986) 'The value of models for care', in B. Kershaw and J. Salvage (eds) *Models for Nursing*, Chichester: John Wiley and Sons.

Meissener, W. W. (1981) 'Metapsychology – who needs it?' *Journal of the American Psychoanalytic Association*, 29: 921.

Meleis, A. I. (1986) 'Theoretical development and domain concepts', in P. Moccia (ed.) *New Approaches to Theory Development*, National League for Nursing.

Merrabeau, L. (1992) 'Tacit nursing knowledge: an untapped resource or a methodological headache?' *Journal of Advanced Nursing*, 17: 108.

Nye, F. I. and Berado, F. N. (1981) *Emerging Conceptual Frameworks in Family Analysis*, London: Macmillan.

Pagana, K. D. (1987) 'Let's stop calling ourselves "patient advocates"', *Nursing*, 2: 51.

Pearson, A. and Vaughan, B. (1986) *Nursing Models for Practice*, Oxford: Heinemann.

Peplau, H. E. (1988) 'The art and science of nursing: similarities, differences and relations', *Nursing Science Quarterly*, 1(1): 8.

Popper, K. R. (1959) *The Logic of Scientific Discovery*, London: Hutchinson.

Reilly, D. E. (1975) 'Why a conceptual framework?' *Nursing Outlook*, 234: 566.

Riehl, J. P. and Roy, C. (1974) *Conceptual Models for Nursing Practice*, Norwalk CT: Appleton-Century-Crofts.

Riehl, J. P. and Roy, C. (1980) *Conceptual Models for Nursing Practice*, 2nd edn, Norwalk; CT: Appleton-Century-Crofts.

Robertson, J. and Robertson, J. (1989) *Separation and the Very Young*, London: Free Association Books.

Sarter, B. (1988) *The Stream of Becoming: a Study of Martha Rogers' Theory*, National League for Nursing.

Schon, D. (1983) *The Reflective Practitioner*, Temple Smith.

Schultz, P. R. (1987) 'When client means more than one: extending the foundational concept of person', *Advances in Nursing Science*, 10(1): 71.

Stainton, M. C. (1982) 'The birth of nursing science', *The Canadian Nurse*, 78(10): 24.

Stanton, M., Paul, C. and Reeves, J. S. (1985) 'An overview of the nursing process', in J. B. George (ed.) *Nursing Theories: the Base for Professional Practice*, Englewood Cliffs, NJ: Prentice-Hall International.

Stevens, B. (1984) *Nursing Theory: Analysis, Application and Evaluation*, 2nd edn, Boston: Little, Brown.

Thibodeau, J. A. (1983) *Nursing Models: Analysis and Evaluation*, Monterey: Wadsworth Health Sciences.

Toffler, A. (1974) *The Psychology of the Future, Learning for Tomorrow*, London: Vintage Books.

Torres, G. (1985) 'The place of concepts and theories within nursing', in J. B. George (ed.) *Nursing Theories: the Base for Professional Nursing Practice*, Englewood Cliffs, NJ: Prentice-Hall International.

Torres, G. and Yura, H. (1974) *Today's Conceptual Framework: its Relationship to the Curricular Development Process*, National League for Nursing.

United Kingdom Central Countil (1992) *Code of Professional Conduct for the Nurse, Midwife and Health Visitor*, 3rd edn, London: UKCC.

Weller, B. (1991) 'An ethnographic study of paediatric practice in an Indian hospital.' Unpublished MSc thesis, Brunel University.

Wright, S. G. (1990) *Building and Using a Model of Nursing*, 2nd edn, London: Edward Arnold.

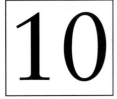

10

THE PROFESSIONS WORKING TOGETHER; LEARNING TO COLLABORATE

Terry Phillips
University of East Anglia

The Need for a Conversational Community to Improve the Quality of Child Care

The Health Service could be likened to a circus. Circuses have a variety of acts which together make up a complete show. Over time, as public values and attitudes change, some of the traditional events disappear and are replaced by other, more appropriate ones, but they always combine to provide a mixture of the familiar and the innovative, the safe and the risky. In the Health Service circus the children's nurses are jugglers, constantly balancing the many and often contradictory demands of care delivery at the uncomfortable interface between the old and the new. They have to carry out their tasks competently within established workplace cultures and institutionalised routines. At the same time, they live and work in a dynamic society which continues to develop its values and strategies with respect to children, families and health. As society becomes increasingly pluralistic, child-care nurses contend with having to act positively within a climate of great uncertainty. As they ride their jugglers' unicycles, they learn to keep their balance by shifting their weight backwards and forwards between safety and risk. At one moment they are calmly and competently carrying out habitual clinical practice which everyone accepts as both safe and appropriate for the particular care needs of the client group. The next moment they are making judgements and taking difficult decisions which are far from risk-free. In a complex society with dynamic (and therefore to some extent unstable) values, judgement is always a matter of the balance of risks. Nurses, because they are professionals, recognise this fact and accept responsibility for making judgements. All too often, however, they are expected to undertake the decision-making process at the centre of their practice without a safety net. To foster the flexibility which enables children's nurses collectively to provide quality care within a context of changing policies, shifting attitudes and inherent risk, individual beliefs and judgements must be kept under scrutiny. For the children's sake, the people who work in child care must talk to one another. Only in the context of a communicative community in which analysis and critique can be developed is it safe to take risks.

From Individual Practical Thinking to Collaborative Reflection on Practice

Mutually educative conversation is integral to professional development in nursing. Nursing is primarily about action, and much of the thinking about practice that children's nurses do takes place in the course of the action itself. It is done by the individual practitioner who, on the spot and without consultation, takes a decision on the evidence immediately available and acts on it. This kind of thinking is described by Carr and Kemmis as *reflection in practice* (Carr and Kemmis, 1987); we might also call it *practical thinking*. The skill which enables practical thinking done in one situation to be built on and used in another is developed outside the area of immediate activity, however, through *reflection on practice*. To move from the status of novice, who assesses each clinical situation as if it were a one-off, to expert, who perceives nursing holistically, requires a paradigm shift (Benner 1984). Experience of as varied a range of practical situations as possible is obviously of importance in bringing this about, but the different way of seeing the world which the term 'paradigm shift' implies is achieved through reflection at a distance from the event. That sort of reflection usually happens in conversation.

The job of the children's nurse is an onerous and complex one. Nursing is a practical profession where competence in 'doing' is of paramount importance. It is also an ethical profession; no nursing activity is without a value position. What makes the task of the individual nurse so testing is the fact that they have to take actions based on their own judgements and decisions in the context of the ethics of their profession and the values of society as a whole. To help children return to wellness as comfortably and speedily as possible they must deploy generic clinical knowledge and nursing skills in very particular ways. In order to provide appropriate care which meets a named child's immediate and particular needs in a specific situation, they must also draw on the 'generic' moral knowledge which is part of society's 'theory' about nursing and about childhood. Without reflection on the values aspect of nursing theory the practice is impoverished, the 'doing' reduced to mere performance, and risk unnecessarily increased. What distinguishes the professional from the non-professional is their level of ability to make judgements and take actions when the unexpected and the ethically problematic arise; this requires a well-thought-out value position. As all the professionals who care for children face similar dilemmas, there is an overwhelming reason for the process of reflection to take place through regular inter-professional dialogue where support and challenge can occur. Unfortunately, however, dialogue, or the sharing of ideas in conversation, has until now taken place mostly in the margins of nursing. A substantial number of nurses regard talking about ideas as of secondary importance to 'getting on and doing'. The truth of the matter is that the two are indivisible in professional practice.

The words 'dialogue' and 'conversation' are ones that any decent thesaurus would locate with 'communication'. It is strange, then, that although the importance of communication in nursing is fully acknowledged, 'dialogue' and 'conversation' rarely appear in texts about it. It is recognised in child-care nursing that the quality of communication with children and relatives is of the essence. It is agreed that while they carry out domestic tasks such as making beds and undertake clinical procedures such as administering drugs, children's nurses must remain alert to the special need a child has for reassurance about separation from their family, and be ready to listen to them and comfort them. It is accepted that while they support the children in the activities of daily living such as dressing and washing themselves, they must talk to them to help them understand their condition. It is also acknowledged that before they can begin to facilitate a child as manager of their own treatment, a nurse must discuss what is involved with the child's family. All these things point to the need for children's nurses to have a high level of communicative competence and to work continually at improving the quality of their communication with both children and their families. But good communication between nurses and children and between nurses and families is

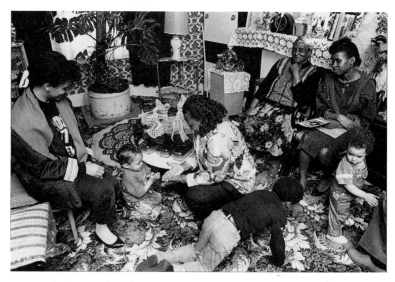

Figure 10.1   Good quality communication with children *and* their families is vital for good quality nursing care

not of itself sufficient to ensure against the temptation to let things slip (without necessarily allowing them to become unsafe) when the maintenance of core values is challenged by circumstances. This will only be assured through conversation with other professionals in a spirit of mutual education towards a critique of practice.

Critical Dialogue as a Means of Challenging the Productivity Myth

If, as has been argued so far, there is a benefit to be had in terms of the improvements in quality of care which can result from nurses discussing with other child-care professionals the pragmatic and value bases of their actions, why are there not more post-event reflective conversations? The answer is hinted at in the metaphors so promiscuously used by Health Service management and government. We are confronted daily by terms like 'purchaser', 'provider', 'delivery' and 'market'. Markets are all about providing what the 'client' needs or wants; they are also about the making of profits to be invested in further business ventures. Because the outcome of time spent talking for *'mutual education towards a critique of practice'* cannot be measured using simplistic, market-related, accountability mechanisms, it is more or less invisible. No one would dispute the value to children of having informed, flexible and proactive nurses looking after them, however, and there is observational evidence that the institutionalisation of colleagual discussion can accelerate a new nurse's progress towards becoming such a practitioner (Phillips *et al.*, 1992; Bedford *et al.*, 1993). There is also observational evidence that without a communicative community in which people talk to one another regularly across professional boundaries, the pressure of daily nursing subverts their intention to practise child-focused nursing (Phillips *et al.*, 1992; Bedford *et al.*, 1993).

A second set of metaphors encapsulate what is happening here. The nurses are asked to balance the need to offer children quality care with the need to attain a specified level of 'throughput', so that the provision of care can be 'cost-effective'. These are the metaphors of manufacturing and mass production, where the means of increasing profit is either to cut staff or increase productivity. Child-care nursing is neither a market nor a manufacturing process; it is a service. Attempts to increase productivity through the extra effort of individual nurses can lead to a breakdown of the service rather than an improvement in it. By working harder, nurses cover up the cracks in the system quite literally at their own expense. Where the managerial and communication structures within hospitals, clinics and other places of work isolate professionals one from the other, individual efforts are resisted by absorbing them. That would most certainly not be cost-effective, and could be downright dangerous for individual children at the point where the breakdown occurs. On the other hand, effort expended on improving clinical practice through collaborative critical dialogue may take pressure away from individual nurses and the children in their care, by affecting practice on a wider scale. Improvement in the quality of care achieved by developing an educative perspective through communication orientated towards analysis, reflection and critique is transformative. In a post-modern era it would be foolish to believe that this sort of collaborative action is likely to change practice beyond the community where the discussion has taken place, but it would be equally unwise to ignore the possibility of change at a local level.

It may be worth illustrating the point just made by offering an example. There are times when a hospitalised child's level of anxiety and trauma are so high that they cannot immediately understand what they are being told or co-operate in the management of their treatment. At times like that there is a high probability that their nurse will have temporarily to neglect the other children in their care to give extra time to them. Whatever additional time the nurse gives, however, it will be difficult to 'consult' the child, or to 'negotiate' with them whilst they are in a state of high anxiety. This situation will be stressful for both the nurse and the child; it will also temporarily increase the strain on the other children from whom attention will be diverted for the time being. Through practical thinking, carried out as the situation unfolds, the nurse may decide to work harder to attend to the remaining children after comforting the first one. Alternatively, again drawing on practical thinking (or reflection in practice) that nurse may choose to back off from any attempt to negotiate with the child and to *impose* a care regime instead. By making the first choice to increase personal productivity as a way of sustaining a workload which cannot easily be managed in the time available when something (mildly) unexpected happens, the nurse may adversely affect their own longer-term health prospects. They will also do nothing to alter the system in which they work to make a similar incident less likely. By choosing the second option, the best interest of the child could be jeopardised. At the time the incident occurs the nurse *must* make a choice; later, however, the decision that led to that choice and the criteria for making the judgement can be the subject of reflection on action. In collaborative discussion with colleagues, where searching or difficult questions can be asked and support given, the nurse can share feelings about the way they dealt with the immediate situation, and explore the value bases of the decisions they made. In the course of looking analytically at what happened, the group can perhaps develop an action plan to improve the future local (namely, workplace area) organisation of care.

From Mere Reflection to Critical Discourse

One of the most important functions of inter-professional communication is that it makes explicit the differences between each profession's beliefs about central care issues and allows the dilemmas created by those differences to be addressed. According to Kress (1985) all discourse is predicated on difference. Another way of putting this is that there is no discourse (theory or belief system), and particularly no professional discourse, in which there are not several competing and sometimes even contradictory subdiscourses. It is impossible not to stand in more than one position. The identity of the child-care nurse is constituted by the discourses of gender, race, childhood and adulthood, and caring, among others. These discourses are in tension: sometimes an issue can look very different when seen from the gender perspective rather than the professional one, for instance. By exploring differences between their own version of what counts as child-care nursing and the version that others hold, members of one group can discover the dilemmas within their own professional rhetoric and the contradictions within their own practice. By exposing the debate (another meaning of the word 'discourse') inherent in professional rhetoric and practices, by exploring the contradictory theories implied by particular forms of practical action and vice versa, and by looking at the way practice and theory influence (or construct) each other, inter-professional discussion can inform the practice of all the groups that take part. Through what Carr and Kemmis call 'committed, interested reflection' (Carr and Kemmis, 1986) groups of child-care professionals can bring together theory and practice in a dialectical relationship which will affect both thought and action in children's nursing. The kind of conversation being referred to is more than chat to exchange information, and more than reflection to describe practice. It is, in fact, critical dialogue. Critical dialogue is defined here as collaborative, analytical discussion about practice which helps to create the general approach to that practice by establishing a climate of critique and an awareness of competing discourses.

Although all professionals know that they work with contradictions, ambiguities and uncertainties, publicly they conspire to maintain a pretence that they have a unified view of their purpose and the means of achieving it. Interviews with Project 2000 nurses about their views on what constitutes competence, for example, show a wide range of interpretations of this core nursing concept (Phillips *et al.*, 1992). It is time the discourse was opened up to professional scrutiny and the implications of difference for action were considered very carefully. To quote Cox *et al.*:

> By reflecting in a committed way we may come to see that many of our deepest beliefs about our nursing worlds may be contradicted in the ways that we think and act; and we may discover that it is not through external forces unrelated to ourselves that we are prevented from meeting our ideals, but the ways we perceive ourselves, our actions, and our worlds. ... Critical reflection exposes ... new ways of knowing and new ways of acting within the world.
>
> (1991: 387)

One of the things that makes a group a profession is its expert knowledge. In an authoritarian culture such as the British one where certainty fosters confidence, the acknowledgement by a particular group that its professional body of knowledge contains unresolved dilemmas can cause the public to doubt its competence. This is yet another reason for children's nurses to meet with their colleagues so that together they can develop the confidence to express their uncertainties and transform their faint unease into a publicly articulated, professional critique of nursing. Such a critique would give children's nurses what Hirschman calls 'voice' (1970; reported in West, 1993). Voice is the means for redressing dissatisfaction through contribution to the debate in the first place and preparation for political action subsequently. Inter-professional exploration of the discourse of child-care nursing can make it apparent that there is no natural or unchallengeable concept involved, and can reveal the areas where there are possibilities for transformative action.

Both reflection in action and reflection on action have the potential to become activities that falsely encourage the person doing the reflecting to think that they have somehow changed things by the act of reflection itself. Without a challenge built into it, reflection can be anodyne. There is little point in reflection on a specific incident in children's nursing simply to describe or give an account of it; the whole purpose of reflecting on an event is to bring it into focus so that it can be analysed. Nurses engaged in the analytical process will examine specific issues in the light of the factors which have shaped them, and in the light of the values which have informed their attitudes towards children and their nursing practice to date. The critique they produce as a consequence of their analysis is likely to be very much more valuable as a basis for future practice than any descriptive account of the event. A reflective professional practitioner without a critique is neither reflective nor professional. But reflective practice with an analytical cutting edge, carried out collaboratively with colleagues who form a critical communicative community, has the power to transform practice.

The move from description to analysis can be achieved quite simply by introducing the question 'why' into the conversation ('Why do we do it that way?', 'Why is that not possible?') (Phillips, 1993a), and adding the speculative 'what if' ('What if we tried this instead?') (Phillips, 1986). By interrogating the taken-for-granted, that is, by asking questions about what has previously seemed axiomatic, and by adopting a hypothetical or exploratory mode of enquiry, learners can discover where the

various discourses which impinge on their work are coming
from (Phillips, 1993b). They will find this much easier to do if
they communicate regularly with people outside their own professional subset because those people will bring slightly different
beliefs and values.

The Problem of Space for Critical Discourse in Hierarchical Networks ———

It has already been suggested that, although critical dialogue
can be a powerful mechanism for changing practice in the community where discussion has taken place, it will not be effective
on an institutional scale. ('Institution' does not necessarily mean
'hospital'; in the sense it is being used here it can mean organisational systems of any kind, including systems for care in the
community.) The mechanisms and structures of large organisations, the Health Service among them, are primarily designed
to ensure the implementation of policy and the assurance of
accountability through a system of line management. Such
structures favour hierarchical communication patterns and
make critical dialogue difficult. Those at the top send messages
downwards; those near the top but not quite at the apex send
messages upwards to their managers and downwards to everyone else. The people at the bottom of the pyramid do not
normally have access to those at the top. In hospitals, service
managers communicate with senior nurses who then communicate with ward sisters, who in turn communicate with their staff
nurses. Staff nurses talk with the sister or charge nurse on their
ward, but rarely to anyone further up the hierarchy. In hierarchical communication systems the top people act as
gatekeepers, and information is only filtered down to others if
the gatekeeper decides it should be. Ideas, critique and practical
perspectives are unable to flow upwards through official channels. This pattern is typical of role cultures (Handy, 1985), like
those found in hospitals and clinics, where people have status
because of the job they do and are communicated with in that
role. Appropriate protocols have to be observed if sanctions are
to be avoided. The *totally* role-culture organisation virtually
precludes democratic critical dialogue, but in most institutions
there are several cultures operating at the same time. The Health
Service is typical in that the role culture predominates, but there
are alternative cultures and communication networks which are
worth seeking out. Where these other cultures operate, and it
is usually at a local level, it is possible for nurses to have space
for critical dialogue as a way of improving care.

Paradoxically, the role-culture structure not only creates top–down communication within nursing, but it also makes inter-professional networking difficult; for even where there is 'sideways' communication from one professional group to another, it is affected by the strength of the hierarchy. The people at the top of one professional group send messages to those at the top of other groups. A nurse manager will either write to (for example) an occupational therapy manager when policy affecting both of them is being formulated or decisions being taken, or will 'discuss' the issue in question with them through a formal agenda at meetings attended by themselves and other managers. It will be far rarer for them to consult colleagues who do the daily work in the other profession; such direct contact with practitioners in another field might seem like an attempt to undermine the managerial position of the senior person in that field. Where a role culture exists, communication between members of one sector and another is usually for the purpose of passing on specialised information related to roles, or for recording (for information only) decisions and actions which a role-holder in one of the sectors has already taken. Within such a structure the opportunity for developing mutual understanding about common issues is limited.

Moving Inter-professional Conversations from the Margins

The scenario described above appears at first to suggest that the possibility of establishing critical communication communities in the Health Service is remote, at least for the nurses and their colleagues who carry out the everyday practice. Hierarchical management structures breed hierarchical communication structures, which in turn discourage the exchange of ideas between professional groups. But successful inter-professional communication does occur. Nurses, social workers, specialist carers, and others bump into one another in the course of a working day and talk to one another about the situation as it unfolds. They have snatched conversations at hand-over times or *ad hoc* chats at odd moments of respite from ongoing busyness. They occasionally meet one another in the restaurant or coffee room, too, where they talk together about the events of the day in an endeavour to make sense of them. These are mostly meetings between pairs of carers, and are unofficial, but they form part of an important alternative communication network that facilitates critical and analytic conversation. Unfortunately, however, by virtue of being unofficial, hurried and private, these conversations are crowded into the margins of nursing practice.

Although conversations in the margins may be the first step on the way to better understanding, there are always pressures on the carers who take part in them to return to 'the job for which they are paid'. This relentless pressure produces a climate in which there is too little time for transforming the beginnings of new understandings into critically informed action. Conversations in the margins can only ever be about peripheral aspects of nursing. Until there is an overwhelming and undeniable demand from ordinary nurses for regular opportunities for participation in inter-professional discussions, the central professional activities of planning and evaluation of care will be done by people other than themselves, particularly doctors, service managers and senior nursing/care staff. Only when there are regular challenges to the dominant discourses of institutionalised child-care nursing will institutions give up saving financial resources by simply *not* providing time. Without challenges, management will, in an adaptation of the American phrase, 'If it ain't broke, don't fix it!', adopt the stance of 'If it ain't damaged so's it notices, let it run until it finally breaks down'. By looking for the spaces where discussion with colleagues can legitimately take place, and then taking the opportunity to see that they do, even the lowest-grade and the most newly qualified children's nurse can begin to improve child-care nursing. 'Local' initiatives using existing communication networks and organisational structures and mechanisms are within the power of the ordinary nurse to achieve in partnership with the ordinary practitioner in the other professions. The six million dollar question, of course, is how to identify where the spaces for those local initiatives are located.

Making a 'Local' Difference

Let us look finally, then, at some possible answers to the question of how to move democratic critical discourse from the margins of child-care nursing to a centre-stage position. This move does not seem likely to happen if ordinary nurses act as if they are independent of the political, economic and cultural context in which they work. Individuals are unlikely to influence either nursing policy or child-care practice through an effort of will, because most organisational cultures resist change. Ironically, when individual child-care nurses work harder to do better what they are already doing, critical conversation is pushed even further into the margins. When the apparent choice is between giving just a bit more time to a child and 'standing around talking' with fellow professionals, there is no contest. It is also the case that most ordinary nurses do not have a direct voice in institutional-level conversations about decision making, judgement, values and resourcing, because critical dialogue of this sort is conducted by senior staff and occurs elsewhere than in the clinical environment. Most organisational cultures institutionalise disempowerment whilst paying lip-service to nursing as an activity which depends upon the quality of nurses as decision makers. If we accept that critical dialogue and the actions which follow from it are two of the things which distinguish professional nursing from other forms of caring, then we must look to places where there is an opportunity for interplay between a focus on the micro-issues of particular clients or specific caring practices, and the macro-issues of policy, resources and values. These points of intersection are all 'local' (that is, within particular environments) and always involve small communities of nurses and their colleagues from supporting professions.

There seem to be three main structures through which the micro and the macro aspects of children's nursing are brought together through discussion which transforms practice. First, there are the quality-assurance structures which exist in all health-care organisations. Secondly, there are the structures for observation and evidence gathering which are an everyday part of nursing. And thirdly, there are the task structures focused on individual children and their carers. Each of these promotes the same pattern of activity and dialogue. A practical problem or issue is identified, evidence collected, discussion and analysis carried out, and further practice initiated. As every nursing environment will have all three structures in place, there is potentially a great deal of opportunity for making a 'local' difference through what is, in essence, the action research process (Elliott, 1991).

Line-management accountability assures quality through extrinsic motivation. A more democratic quality assurance takes place whenever a task group (such as those we find in formally constituted primary nursing and community-care teams, but which can also be composed of informal teams of professionals who have a specific task to do) meet to talk about a particular child or group of children. Its motivation is entirely intrinsic and encourages an interplay between talk about the micro-issues of assuring quality of care for particular children, and talk about the macro-issues of policy, resources and values which also affect the quality of care. The development of a 'local' culture in which nursing itself is examined alongside particular practice depends upon the setting up of an educative agenda. Such an agenda is created when nurses, physiotherapists, occupational therapists and others hold team meetings to discuss a particular child's case.

A team of two or three who meet regularly can begin to challenge some of the assumptions behind one another's clinical practice. Because it is aimed at improving care for particular children in specific circumstances, and is a matter of concern to the team as a whole, this sort of critical dialogue is obviously relevant to immediate practice and is therefore more likely to affect the future practice of the team. In discussing an issue or problem arising directly from practice, individuals can ask *'why?'* and explore alternatives through *'what if?'* questions. When making a claim or suggestion, members of a team can expect to offer relevant observational evidence, and anyone wishing to challenge an assumption behind a claim could expect to offer counter or modifying evidence. In this way the team would begin to draw up their own theory of children's nursing. They would move away from the approach to theory which treats it as something which is 'in the literature' and so has either to be treated with great respect ignored, or 'translated' from out there into practice. They would continue to focus on practice, but would expect as a team to critique it and change it through collaborative conversations in the workplace. Teams who provide a little time for critical dialogue create 'local' differences in the quality of care by placing the professional competences of gathering, analysing and evaluating evidence centre-stage in child-care nursing.

References

Bedford, H., Phillips, T., Robinson, J. and Schostak, J. (1993) *Assessment of Competeness in Nursing and Midwifery Education and Training*, Norwich, Centre for Applied Research in Education, University of East Anglia, and Sheffield, English National Board for Nursing, Midwifery and Health Visiting.

Benner, P. (1984) *From Novice to Expert: Excellence and Power in Clinical Nursing Practice*, California: Addison-Wesley.

Carr, W. and Kemmis, S. (1983) *Becoming Critical: Knowing through Action Research*, Geelong: Deakin University Press.

Cox, H., Hickson, P. and Taylor, B. (1991) 'Exploring reflection: knowing and constructing practice', in G. Gray and R. Pratt (eds) *Towards a Discipline of Nursing*, London: Churchill Livingstone.

Elliott, J. (1991) *Action Research for Educational Change*, Milton Keynes: Open University Press.

Handy, C. (1985) *Understanding Organisations*, 3rd edn. Harmondsworth: Penguin Business.

Hirschman, P. (1970) reported in West, S. (1993) *Educational Values for School Leadership*, London: Kogan Page.

Kress, G (1985) *Linguistic Processes in Sociocultural Practice*, Geelong: Deakin University Press.

Phillips, T. (1986) 'Beyond lip-service: discourse development after the age of nine' in B. Mayor and A. Pugh (eds) *Language, Communication, and Learning*, London: Croom Helm (in association with the Open University).

Phillips, T. (1992a) '"Why?" the neglected question in curriculum planning' in K. Norman (ed.) *Thinking Voices*, London: Longman (in association with the National Oracy Project).

Phillips, T. (1993b). 'The dead spot in our struggle for meaning: learning and understanding through small group talk', in D. Wray (ed.) *Teaching Primary English: the State of the Art*.

Phillips, T., Schostak, J., Bedford, H. and Robinson, J. (1992) *The Assessment of Competencies in Nurse and Midwife Education and Training (Interim Report)*, Norwich: Centre for Applied Research in Education, University of East Anglia.

West, S. (1993) *Educational Values for School Leadership*, London: Kogan Page.

<table>
11
</table>

THE CONTINUUM OF CARE

Jayne Taylor
Suffolk College

Provision of health services for children and their families has been the focus of much criticism since the inception of the National Health Service in 1948. The failure of both community and hospital services to respond effectively to new knowledge about the complex needs of children and their families has been the theme of much expert and lay investigation and research. Although improvements have been noted in some areas, there still remains a wealth of knowledge that has not been acted on.

This chapter looks at the continuum of child health care and analyses many extant community and hospital facilities for children, highlighting the need to ensure that child health services are integrated and offer satisfaction to the consumer. Although it has not been possible to look at every service involved in the care of children, it is hoped that the discussion here will give the reader a critical overview of care provision for children and encourage health-care professionals to reconceptualise existing practices.

Hospital Services for Children and Their Families

National Health Service provision for children has undergone major reform over the last forty years. This has been partially due to greater awareness that long periods of separation from parents could have long-term detrimental effects on the psychological development of children (Bowlby, 1953; Robertson and Robertson, 1989). The Platt Report (1959) reiterated the findings of these psychologists by recommending that children should only be admitted to hospital if absolutely necessary and that children had the right to be cared for by suitably qualified staff. The National Association for the Welfare of Children in Hospital (NAWCH) – now renamed Action for Sick Children – has unceasingly campaigned for the rights of children and for health-care professionals to respond to the recommendations of Platt.

Two Consumers' Association reports (1980, 1985) investigated the extent to which the earlier Platt Report recommendations had been acted upon. The first report was highly critical of existing services, finding that many children were being cared for on adult wards and were deprived of their parents' presence, often for several days at a time if they were in hospital for surgery. The second report showed that the situation had improved during the early 1980s with fewer children being cared for on adult wards, more wards adopting open visiting policies and more offering facilities for resident parents. The improvement was, however, not universal. Furthermore, Action for Sick Children was bringing to the fore new problems experienced by children and their families. The facilities for resident parents, the attitude of nurses towards parents, the plight of children in other hospital departments, the difficulties experienced by adolescents and the preparation of children for hospitalisation are but a few of the areas that have been criticised. A more recent report (Department of Health, 1991) has taken account of the Action for Sick Children campaigns and has made recommendations relating to children's services. The cardinal principles of this report reiterate the need for high standards of care, family access, avoiding admission (or discharging children early) whenever possible, parental participation in care, separate child facilities with separate adolescent facilities wherever possible, the rights of the child in relation to privacy, and information appropriate to the age and understanding of the child. The needs of sick children in hospital do, however, vary according to their age and conceptual development, the onset, severity and duration of their illness, as well as other complex psychosocial influences. The next section looks at the care of children and their families in acute hospital areas.

Children in the operating department _____

Many children are admitted to hospital for routine and emergency surgery each year. Their needs before, during and following surgery are complex, and if, as health-care professionals, we fail to recognise and meet these needs the long-term emotional effects on the child can be potentially severe (Radford, 1990; Smallwood, 1988).

For children being admitted for routine surgery, either as day patients or as in-patients, there are many ways in which parents, nurses and other professionals can intervene to minimise the emotional effects of the child's experience. Many hospitals now offer pre-admission visits to children and their families so that they can familiarise themselves, to some extent, with the hospital environment and hospital routine. The quality and content of pre-admission visiting varies, however, with some hospitals offering a quick look around the ward areas whilst others organise visits to the theatre for those who wish, have play therapy sessions where children can play with dolls in theatre dress, ride on theatre trolleys and become familiar with some of the equipment utilised in theatre (Smallwood, 1988; Bates and Broome, 1986). Other units are experimenting with the use of videos and booklets as a way of preparing children for hospitalisation, as well as evening visits for parents who can assimilate information without distraction, and more reliably reinforce the information given to their children during their own pre-admission visit.

There is, without doubt, a need to evaluate the effectiveness of any innovation, and this is particularly important in the area of pre-admission visiting, which aims to lower anxiety. One such evaluation was undertaken by Marriner (1988) in a small study in Jersey. Although the research has several limitations, it was able to give support to the view that specific pre-hospital preparation can 'assist in uncomplicated and smoother postoperative recovery'. Bates and Broome (1986), however in their excellent review of research into children undergoing surgery, identify the need for further research, particularly into the content and timing of pre-admission visits in relation to several variables, including age, developmental ability, previous experiences, parental responses and nursing care.

Clearly, not all children will be able to attend for a pre-admission visit to hospital – for example, children who are admitted for emergency surgery or who cannot visit because of distance or domestic limitations. These children are equally at risk of the potential emotional trauma of undergoing surgery, and each department should develop a policy to ensure that their needs are not overlooked. Parents who cannot visit, for whatever reason, should be encouraged to contact the ward if they have any worries, and specific information should be sent to the family about appropriate physical and psychological

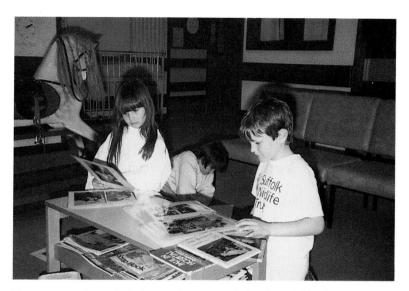

Figure 11.1   Pre-admission visiting can help the child's post-operative recovery

preparation. Colliss (1990) identified, for example, that a particular area of concern is pre-operative fasting for children admitted on the day of operation. Each ward should also have age-specific resources, such as books, leaflets and dolls, for children admitted as emergencies, so they can be given relevant information, if their condition allows, during the time between admission and surgery.

Most children who undergo surgery have a general anaesthetic, but the time between arriving in the theatre suite and the induction of anaesthesia can be traumatic for the child (Perthen, 1990). There has been a move over the last decade towards encouraging one parent to accompany a child to the anaesthetic room, although the practice is by no means universal. A study by the British Association of Paediatric Anaesthetists (cited in Coulson, 1988) showed that only 55 per cent of anaesthetists supported parental presence. Glasper (1991), reporting on an unpublished survey of anaesthetists undertaken by Glasper and Dewar in 1986, highlighted a 'dichotomy of opinion', and suggested that further investigation would help to 'unmask the confusion' that exists in relation to opinions and practices among anaesthetists.

Since Glasper and Dewar's study (Glasper, 1991) there have been studies which have attempted to investigate the benefits of parental presence in the anaesthetic room (Perthen, 1990;

Coulson, 1988). Coulson's study used observation and interview techniques to measure the effectiveness of parental presence. She found that parents were not disruptive, that 91 per cent of the children remembered the parent's presence when going to sleep, and that parents felt it was helpful to be present. However, 20 per cent of parents felt that their presence made no difference to their child, and 6.7 per cent felt that their presence had made things worse. Clearly, further investigation is necessary to identify if there are instances when it may be preferable for the parents not to accompany their child. Until that time, the evidence suggests that it is usually beneficial for both parents and children if they can remain together until the child is asleep.

Following surgery, one of the most important factors in minimising trauma is the effective control of pain and vomiting. Radford (1990) suggests that pain and vomiting are better prevented than treated, and that the first dose of analgesia is best administered whilst the child is still asleep. Continuous infusions of analgesia are more effective than bolus dosages. Colliss (1990) also suggests that patient-controlled analgesia may be used for some children.

Eland (1988) has been undertaking research into pain control in children for nearly twenty years and has highlighted several important areas of concern. First, there is a need to consider the child's knowledge of pain. In one of Eland's early studies, it was found that over half of the children studied did not know the meaning of the word 'pain'. Secondly, the way in which analgesics are prescribed is important. Eland found that children who were prescribed *prn* analgesia were not given it even when they had pain. Eland suggests that alternative ways of prescribing and administering pain control may be more appropriate. Thirdly, Eland found that there was an inverse relationship between the amount of time parents spent with their child and the frequency with which the child received analgesia. Eland hypothesised that parental comfort may minimise fear and anxiety, thus decreasing pain. Finally, there is a need to develop and use appropriate measuring tools to assess pain levels in children and the effectiveness of analgesia. Eland has developed the Eland Color Tool which measures qualitative and quantitative aspects of pain in young children. Other pain assessment tools have been developed for use with other age groups of children such as verbal scales, visual analogue scales, faces, poker chips, 'X' marks the spot and pain diaries (see Alder, 1991).

The parent's help in minimising the effects of surgery is an important aspect of post-operative recovery. Parents are usually very familiar with their child's behaviour patterns, fears, anxieties and language skills. Nurses can use parental skills to give information to the child about specialised equipment, medical and nursing interventions and pain control.

Children in intensive care

Children vary in their ability to understand illness and treatment. However, Oskala and Merenmies (1989) suggest that the vast majority of children find it more difficult than adults to cope with the intensive care unit because of their 'age, stage of development and limited experiences in crisis situations'. Their study, which looked at human needs in children admitted to intensive care, following open heart surgery units suggested that as children progress through their stay in intensive care their needs will change. The data, which were gathered by the nurses in intensive care, showed that the need for 'rest and leisure' was constant throughout the child's stay, but that needs such as 'safety and tenderness' became important after the initial 'survival' problems had passed.

Fradd (1986) also discusses the needs of children in intensive care and the importance of maintaining some semblance of normality in the child's world. Intensive care can appear to be a totally hostile environment to the child, so familiar people and objects are extremely important to them. Parental presence, favourite toys and books may help the child to orientate and be distracted. Fradd describes how in one hospital, school-age children with head injuries and those who have had neurosurgery are visited by teachers whilst they are still in intensive care, which provides the child with stimulation and is something familiar to them.

The needs of parents and other members of the family should also be identified and met by those health-care professionals involved in intensive care. A recent study by Rukholm *et al.* (1991) identified that families needed to be assured that their relatives were receiving the best care as well as receiving honest information about care, prognosis and progress. Parents should be encouraged to participate actively in basic care and can be taught to participate in more skilled procedures. Staff should, however, acknowledge that families need to rest, eat and have some time to themselves, and can help parents by ensuring that they are called if a child's condition changes, or if the child asks for a parent. Social service assistance can be requested, if the parents wish, so that siblings can be looked after, allowing parents to be with their sick child.

The British Paediatric Association Working Party on Paediatric Intensive Care (1987) found that many critically ill children are cared for in adult intensive care units, where the majority of patients are adults. In this situation it is important that nursing and medical staff segregate children, as far as possible, from adult patients and make every effort to ensure that the environment is appropriate for a child. The Department of Health (1991) advises that whether children are cared for in designated paediatric intensive care units or within a designated area of an adult unit, certain standards should be adhered to. These include the following:

1 the nurse in charge should be a qualified first-level children's nurse and should preferably have undertaken further training in intensive care;
2 facilities should be available for parents/carers to remain with their children and they should participate in their care if appropriate;
3 play facilities should be available under the supervision of a play specialist, for those children who would derive benefit from them.

Children in the accident and emergency department

The accident department is often the first contact that many children have with hospitals, and it has been estimated that about 3 million children attend hospital accident and emergency departments each year (NAWCH, 1990), and that a third of all patients seen in accident and emergency departments are children (Department of Health, 1991).

Although some hospitals offer specialist accident and emergency facilities for children, many provide a shared facility for both children and adults. Any health-care professional who has worked in an accident and emergency department will be familiar with some of the horrific sights that can cause both concern and anxiety to adults, and it is important that children attending the department, whether as patients or visitors, are not subjected to experiences which may cause them distress. The environment should be as child-friendly as possible, with separate waiting areas and treatment facilities which are bright and cheerful, with a good range of washable toys and books which can be used to distract children during their time in the department (Mead, 1991). Any child who has been suddenly injured will be frightened and confused, and parents frequently experience a range of emotions, from guilt, extreme anxiety and fear, to loss of control. Inevitably, the immediate physical needs of the child must take priority, but it is also important that the psychological needs of the child and family are assessed and appropriate interventions are offered. Nursing staff who are trained and experienced in the care of children should be assigned to care for children and their families in the department. Knowledge of child development and how to communicate with children of all ages is a necessity for effective care.

Information about investigations and possible treatment should be given to both parents and children, and questions answered in an honest way, free from jargon. Parents should have access to examination rooms, X-ray suites and anaesthetic rooms so that they can be involved in care and help the child through any potentially frightening experiences (Department of Health, 1991). In some cases – for example, road traffic accidents – parents may also be in need of treatment, and nursing staff should ensure that at least parents and children are kept informed of the progress of each other. It is preferable, if the physical needs of both allow it, that such parents and children should not be separated.

There are two groups of children for whom special consideration should be given in the accident and emergency department. The first group are children and adolescents who have, or it is suspected that they may have, harmed themselves deliberately. Steinberg (1987) suggests that any threat or hint of suicide should always be taken seriously. These children need special help, and referral to the child psychiatric team is frequently necessary (see Circular HN(84)25/LASS(84)5 – *Health Service Management: the Management of Deliberate Self Harm*). Whilst the child is in the accident department, nursing staff should make every effort to *listen* to what the child is saying, as this information may be invaluable to the later care of the child. Nurses should be particularly sensitive to the child's wishes about, for example, seeing parents. On the other hand, parents should be kept informed about what is happening to the child and may be able to provide information about the child's emotional state leading up to the attempted self-harm.

The second group of children who need special consideration are those where it is known, or suspected, that the child has been deliberately harmed by the parent. Nurses in the accident department inevitably spend more time with the child and family than other health workers, and it is often the nurse who picks up clues about the nature of the injury which lead to suspicion and subsequent investigations. Wailes (1983) suggests that any doubt about the child's injury, or the parents' behaviour, should be communicated to medical staff or senior nursing staff. Nursing staff involved with children in the accident department should receive special training in the recognition of child abuse and should be aware of where they can obtain specialist advice (Department of Health, 1991). Each department should have a defined policy for the care of children in need of protection.

Finally, to conclude this section on the accident and emergency department, discharge planning should be considered. Most children and parents will be distressed following their visit to the department, and even if the injury is relatively minor, may go home to face recrimination and accusations from each other, members of their immediate and extended family and other parties, including, in some instances, the police. It is important that the aftercare of the child is not neglected amongst all this emotional turmoil, so discharge information should be clear and instructions written down in a form that parents and/or the child will be able to understand. The general practitioner should be notified of any treatment instigated and follow-up care needed (Department of Health, 1991).

Children admitted to hospital wards

The general philosophy of the child health services has been to reduce the time spent by children in hospital to a minimum in order to prevent the short- and long-term detrimental effects of hospitalisation (Caring for Children in the Health Services Committee, 1988). Other innovations have also been instrumental in changing the nature of a child's experience of hospital, such as shared care with parents, care-by-parents units, the move towards primary nursing, and the recognition that children should be cared for in specially designated departments under the auspices of suitably qualified health-care workers. Many of these innovations resulted from research with children, whilst others, such as the concept of the named nurse, can be attributed to a greater awareness of the needs of all patients in hospital.

The admission procedure is one area that has caused concern to many. Glen (1982), writing about admission, suggests that it is a procedure that not only first introduces the child to the ward, but can also influence the child's subsequent experience of hospital. Nurses should never view admission as routine but should be aware of the physical, psychological, cultural and social needs of the child and family. A comprehensive assessment based around a framework recognised by all health workers involved in care should be undertaken and opportunity given for the family and the child to ask questions. Burr (1990) suggests that the children, especially older children and adolescents, should be interviewed on their own as well as with parents because they may wish to discuss specific problems in confidence or areas of concern which parental presence may inhibit. The admission interview is an opportune time for information giving, especially if the child and family have been unable to attend for a pre-admission visit. The Department of Health (1991) suggests that information which is age-appropriate should be given in a culturally sensitive way about the reasons for admission, the proposed treatment and its significant side-effects and prognosis, the name of the consultant, facilities for resident parents, toys, clothes and the expected duration of the hospitalisation. Wherever possible, admission should be undertaken by a suitably qualified nurse, and recognition given by ward managers that the admission procedure is a skilled activity which should not be underemphasised.

Whilst children are in hospital, their lives are liable to be a constant round of investigations, procedures and therapeutic interventions. Inevitably children will be required to interact with many different professionals who have specific roles to play in child and family care. Fradd (1987) discusses the need to ensure that care is well co-ordinated and that all those involved in the child's care work as a team which 'utilizes each professional's skills, facilitates and supports staff members, and recognizes each discipline's accountability to the quality and care given to children and their families'. The team will of course consist of nurses who are involved with the care of the child and family during their stay in hospital. Rodin (1983) discusses reports of a child in an orthopaedic hospital who had no fewer than twenty-three complete changes in staff during her hospitalisation. Clearly, interaction with such large numbers of nurses is inadvisable, particularly when the child is ill and may have a reduced capacity for making new relationships (Muller *et al.*, 1992). Weller (1980) suggests that nurses should be encouraged to become familiar with a few children, or in some instances, one child, rather than engage in a series of tasks which brings them into contact with all children on a ward.

Individualising care in this way will bring benefits to the nurse, the child and the family, who are able to form a closer relationship with one another (Hall, 1987; Brown, 1989).

The presence of parents can help to minimise the distress felt by children, and research over the last thirty years has shown that the presence of a familiar person can help the child to cope better with the experience of hospitalisation (Caring for Children in the Health Services Committee, 1988). This need is often greater at night, because, whereas many children are used to being away from parents during the day, they are not used to being separated at night. The Caring for Children in the Health Services Committee's report (1988) suggests that beds should be provided for one parent in the following proportions:

- for all under 5-year-olds;
- for 75% of 5–7-year-olds;
- for 50% of 8–11-year-olds; and
- for 25% of 12–16 year olds.

Parents who cannot stay at night, for whatever reason, should not be made to feel guilty and should be given assurances that they will be contacted at home if necessary.

Whilst parents are with their children they should be actively encouraged to participate in those aspects of care which they feel confident and competent to undertake. In some instances this care will be very basic, but many parents are taught to undertake more complex care, particularly if the care will be ongoing after the discharge of the child. For some children with chronic illness, parents may have already been taught to carry out high-level skills prior to hospitalisation and may in some cases be more knowledgeable about the child's condition than many of the nursing staff (Muller *et al.*, 1992). Regardless of the extent to which parents are involved in care, the care plan should clearly record what aspects of care are to be carried out by each individual. This will prevent confusion for the child and will help clarify the roles of all those involved in care.

Finally, it is important to mention the environment. It is widely advocated that children admitted to hospital should be nursed on children's wards by nurses trained in the care of children (Department of Health, 1991). However, research undertaken by the Consumers' Association (1985) showed that this is not always the reality. A further problem is the marked lack of adolescent units where young people can be cared for by nurses who are sensitive to their special needs (Muller *et al.*, 1992). Surely, it is time for health authorities to look critically at the services they provide and take note of the guidance offered by statutory and voluntary bodies in relation to the needs of children and young people in hospital.

Community Services for Children and Their Families

It is sometimes forgotten by those involved in the care of children in hospital that the majority of sick children are successfully cared for at home by their families, with or without the support of community-based health-care professionals. The general practitioner has for many years been at the forefront of providing primary medical care for sick children, enabling children who may in previous times have been admitted to hospital to remain at home to be cared for by their natural carers. The general practitioner service is, in theory, available to all and free at the point of access. Prentice (1991) writes in her paper on Health Service reform:

> in terms of equity of access, the present system of primary medical care in Britain has achieved major successes. Regardless of where you live in the country or your level of income or education, access to primary medical care at general practitioner level is virtually guaranteed for all client groups.

There is, however, evidence that the view held by Prentice does not show the true picture of the state of health care, particularly in relation to child health. The Black Report (1980) is one of the most comprehensive accounts of inequality in health-care provision in Britain, supporting the view that low social class and lack of education can be barriers which prevent equal access to health care. Culture and race can also affect both access to and provision of primary medical care. Taylor (1991) discusses the plight of travellers, who either find their access to general practitioner services is barred by bureaucracy, or that services on offer are so ethnocentric that they are unacceptable to their beliefs and traditions. Currer (1991) and Watson (1991) also discuss access and client satisfaction in their respective studies of Pathan and Bengali families in Britain. Currer (1991) warns that health-care workers should guard against racism within their practice, and highlights three common characteristics of racist work: the concentration on cultural explanations as a way of explaining behaviours; the failure of health-care workers to examine the cultural 'underpinnings' of health care; and unequal power of interaction. The importance of this research is to highlight the need to ensure that clients' perspectives are not only understood and respected, but also that account is taken of cultural needs when planning services.

Primary medical care in Britain is undergoing great change as a result of the NHS and Community Care Act (1990), and there are doubts as to whether the actual and proposed changes will improve the health of children (Prentice, 1991; Potrykus, 1991). General practitioners are being encouraged to become budget-holders, although this move was initially limited to large practices. The reality of what this may mean to families, as well as community nurses, practice nurses, midwives and health visitors, has been the focus of some speculation. Children who have chronic or serious ill-health problems may, in future, be unattractive to general practitioners who have to keep within their allocated budgets (Willcox, 1990). The cost, for example, of referring a child with cancer to a 'centre of excellence' may be so great that the general practitioner could refuse the family access to their practice list.

The quality of care for ill children is not the only area of doubt in the current political climate. The NHS and Community Care Act (1990) offers financial incentives for general practitioners to undertake preventive health care. The incentives are paid on the basis of reaching minimum and maximum targets for immunisation as well as for other secondary and tertiary preventive services, such as child health surveillance. However, the emphasis is placed on quantifiable services and little recognition is given to other important and often time-consuming aspects of the general practitioner's role. There are also fears that general practitioners will delegate many of their preventive services to practice nurses, who are not trained to undertake them. Norman (1991) discusses the dramatic increase in practice nurses employed by general practitioners which gives rise, she suggests, to 'concerns about training, supervision and quality of care'. If a comprehensive preventive service for children is to be offered by general practitioners, they must be prepared to employ children's nurses and acknowledge that child health surveillance is a skill which requires, amongst other things, an ability to communicate with children and a knowledge of normal child development. If general practitioner services for children emerge as a 'task and target' service it will surely be to the ultimate detriment of all but the child's physiological well-being.

Health visiting

The NHS and Community Care Act (1990) has, without doubt, wide-reaching implications for existing health visiting services, as does the implementation of Project 2000 which will educate child nurses to be competent to care in both hospital and community settings. Many health visitors fear that their role is being eroded by general practitioners, practice nurses, paediatric community nurses and the new Project 2000 child nurses. We can only wait and see how profound the effects of the NHS and Community Care Act and Project 2000 will be, although Potrykus (1991) fears that 'the UKCC's "nurse practitioners" and the rise of the practice nurse seem to be edging out health visiting as an autonomous profession'.

The role of the health visitor in the prevention of ill health and in health promotion has had important and measurable success. Apart from midwives and to a lesser extent school nurses, health visitors have been the only health-care professionals to be routinely involved with all children and families, regardless of their health status.

There has been, however, and still is, some controversy about the role of health visitors. One of the main problems, according to Clark (1973), was that there was 'a dearth of factual information about the content of the ... work of the health visitor'. The debate about what health visitors actually do has continued to the present day, with some professionals and members of the public displaying poor understanding of their role. A survey carried out by Crabbe (1988) looked at public perceptions of the health visitor's role and found several misconceptions and some very bizarre perceptions. Several respondents confused the roles of midwives, social workers and even educational welfare workers with that of the health visitor. Clark (1984), in her research, also found that consumers of the service did not understand what the health-visiting service did and what it was for.

The picture is not, however, entirely negative, and more recent research into health-visiting practice has been carried out with encouraging results. Weatherley (1988) undertook a survey of client satisfaction, and found that there was 'quite a high level of satisfaction with the service'. This survey also found that the health visitor's concentration on the 0- to 1-year-olds was well justified and met consumer need. This point was further emphasised by another survey carried out by Duncan *et al.* (1986) who set up an out-of-hours service in Scotland. The researchers found that out of a total of 2,488 calls over a two-year period the vast majority of calls were for children in their first year, with calls for 0- to 3-month babies scoring most frequently. Another study by Powell (1986) in Gosport confirmed the findings of the earlier 'Sheffield study' (Battye and Deaken, 1979) that an intensive home infant surveillance system could have a significant impact on improving care and infant mortality. This proactive approach to the health of children in response to epidemiological data is without doubt the way forward for the health-visiting service.

Further studies (Gastrell, 1986; Husain, 1990) suggested that clients also found child health clinics to be valuable. Gastrell found that clients perceived monitoring of their child's height and weight, confirmation of their progress, talking to health visitors about their children and advice about particular problems to be the most useful aspects of this service. Sherratt *et al.* (1991), in their study of parental concern, found that 90 per cent of mothers in their sample attended child health clinics and also found that one of the main reasons for attending was for baby weighing. Another interesting implication of this research was the suggestion that there may be a need for health visitors to have more training in the 'diagnosis and management of minor ailments which are of such major concern to mothers'.

This discussion of the health-visiting service as part of the continuum of child care would be incomplete if it failed to mention the negative views held by some clients in relation to the service. Foster and Mayall (1990), in their study of health visitors as health educators, conclude that 'mothers in this and other studies confirm that some health visitors do behave in ways they find unacceptable'. Sefi (1988) found in her research into verbal exchanges during the health visitor's first visit to the mother's home that health visitors tended to work within a framework which was 'a task based, problem solving medical model'. This 'top-down' approach has been shown to be ineffective and unpopular with mothers, who prefer health visitors to respond sensitively to individual need (Foster and Mayall, 1990).

In this section, the lack of clear understanding by consumers about the role of the health visitor has been highlighted and studies of client satisfaction have been discussed. What is clear is that health visitors have a role and function with families and young children but that this role needs to be clarified and extended. In the climate of change, health visitors must use research evidence even if it requires a radical reorganisation of their working practice. Inevitably, if health visitors do not steer in the direction of change, other health-care professionals will do it for them.

The school nursing service has a long history and has undergone frequent change and reform. From the early days when the school nurses' main role was 'as receptionists to the doctors and as hunters of vermin' (Vine, 1991), their place in caring for the holistic needs of children during their time in school has become firmly established. The NHS and Community Care Act (1990) has to some extent removed some of the mundane tasks traditionally carried out by school nurses, such as immunisation. The onus of this facet of the school nurse's role has now largely been placed with the general practitioner. As a result many school nurses are able to develop their role as promotors of health and health educators, both on an individual and a group basis.

When the school health service was incorporated in the NHS in 1974, school medicals were no longer a statutory requirement and the number of medicals carried out after initial school entry declined. However, the Court Report (1976) and the Hall Report (1989) questioned the value of undertaking even these routine school entry medicals, and many areas are reviewing their policies in the light of such expert reports. Ealing Health Authority is an example of one authority which has introduced a new school health programme aimed to cut out the routine and often unnecessary school medicals during early schooling (Mattock, 1991). Holt (1990) describes a system in Southampton where all 11-year-olds undergo a health appraisal system rather than a traditional medical assessment. This system has five objectives:

1   to provide a health profile of each schoolchild;
2   to provide a health profile for each school;
3   to allow children to discuss their health needs as perceived by them;
4   to increase teacher participation in health issues; and
5   to consider alternative working methods for school nurses in order to allow them to develop and use specialist skills.

The need for the school health service to adapt to the needs of schoolchildren is paramount, and Pippa Bagnall, in a interview with Jackson (1991), reiterated the need for school nurses to target health needs and develop health profiles. Bagnall also discusses the potential for school nurses to develop expertise, possibly with children of different ages. The health needs of adolescents in a secondary school are, for example, very different from those of younger children. School nurses working

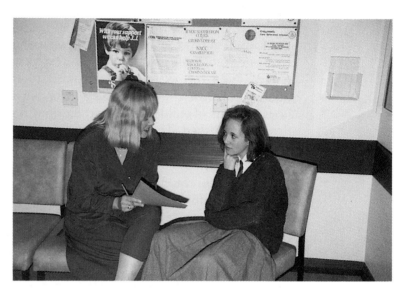

Figure 11.2   The role of the nurse with adolescents needs both knowledge of developmental theory and counselling skills

with adolescents require particular expertise in counselling as well as a working knowledge of the psychosocial and emotional theories of adolescent development.

There is also a role for school nurses to play in group health education in the classroom, although Bagnall (in Jackson, 1991) warns that the school nurse's input should be in addition to that of the teacher rather than as a replacement. It is also important that the nurses are seen as separate from the education system so that they do not discourage pupils with problems from consulting them. School nurses should be part of the school rather than an infrequent visitor who comes in to undertake a series of mechanistic tasks. Regular 'drop-in surgeries' have been successful in many schools, with the nurse taking a client-directed approach to health promotion.

Paediatric community nursing

Advances in medical and nursing care, and an increase in hospital day surgery, have resulted in many children with acute and chronic health needs spending less time in hospital, thus avoiding the detrimental effects of hospitalisation. In order to meet the needs of these children and their families, several health authorities have set up paediatric community nursing teams (Whiting, 1989). These teams enable children to avoid unnecessary overnight stays in hospital and in many areas enable families to have a realistic choice about where children with life-threatening illnesses spend their remaining time (Atwell and Gow, 1985). Glasper *et al.* (1989) also discuss the valuable role that community teams can play with the family after the death of a child.

Community children's nursing teams rely on effective communication between all health-care workers involved in the care of the family and the child (Fradd, 1987; Kitson *et al.*, 1987). Failure can result, usually because of inadequate family resources and a lack of communication (Harris, 1988), leaving families and professionals feeling guilty and anxious. It is important, therefore, that both the nurses and the families concerned should have the right to request, and gain, access to hospital care if they feel it is in the best interests of the child and family.

The advantages of remaining at home for the child and family are many, particularly if the child has a chronic health problem which may previously have resulted in frequent visits to hospital for intravenous medication, physiotherapy, wound dressings and other interventions. For the child, less time lost from school and less time spent away from the family and friends are obvious consequences. There are also benefits for the other members of the family. An early qualitative study by Hayes and Knox (1984) highlighted the disruptions that occurred to the lives of families when a child had a long-term health problem requiring frequent periods of hospitalisation. Siblings are also affected, and Craft and Wyatt (1986), who studied a group of siblings of children hospitalised for chronic health problems, found that siblings experienced increased nervousness and had difficulty in sleeping. Clearly, many of these problems can be avoided if the ill child can remain at home with the support of an appropriately qualified, autonomous child-care nurse.

The concept of paediatric community nursing care is not restricted to older babies, children and adolescents but also applies to neonates. There is still a great deal of controversy about early bonding and its long-term consequences, but even at birth the infant's senses are all functional to some degree and they are, according to Haith (1986), 'much more than mere recipients of environmental stimuli'. Furthermore, Couriel and Davies (1988), in their view of research relating to babies who have required prolonged admission to neonatal intensive care units, discuss the frequent readmission rates, the increased risk of sudden infant death, failure to thrive and non-accidental injury and difficulties in parent and child relationships. Extending community paediatric nursing care to encompass very low birth weight and premature babies is justifiable in view of these potential problems. Couriel and Davies found, in their study of one such service in Manchester, that early discharge into the community with support from specialist nurses is advantageous to the families and the neonate. Few babies need to be readmitted, pressure on existing intensive care cots was relieved and the service was estimated to be cost-effective.

Children with severe learning disabilities in the community

The care of children with severe learning disabilities has changed dramatically over the last two decades, with the emphasis being on community care and avoiding, at all costs, children growing up in large mental handicap hospitals. The 1989 Department of Health report *Caring for People* recommended that children with special needs should only be admitted to hospital if they required acute care which could not be provided by the primary health-care team.

The move towards community care has had inevitable implications for both health-care professionals and the families involved. There may be many professionals involved in the lives of families, offering a range of health, social and educational services designed to enable each child to reach full potential and to give maximum family support. It is of vital importance that these workers communicate effectively with one another so that services are neither duplicated nor omitted. For example, it is possible that the nursing input alone may consist of the health visitor, the school nurse, the paediatric community nurse and the community mental handicap nurse. Collaboration and negotiation with the family is paramount from the time at which the problem is suspected, through the assessment process and continuing as the child grows up. The needs of families caring for a child with severe learning disabilities are not constant, and health-care professionals working in the community should be sensitive to change. Hirose and Veda (1990), in their study of children with cerebral palsy and the coping behaviour of parents, found that 'crisis periods' occurred throughout the child's life, with the most stressful periods being around the time of diagnosis, followed by toddlerhood, schooling, adolescence and when their child reached adulthood. The study found that whilst mothers undertook the major responsibility for care, fathers were the most important source of support for mothers. A further study by Carr (1988) identified a similar picture in a study of families caring for a child with Down's syndrome. She found that parents were frequently affected both psychologically and physiologically, but that it was the mothers who had higher morbidity than other members of the family. Carr (1988) also noted that siblings can be affected but that variables such as age, sex, position in the family, the number of children in the family, socio-economic class and parental attitudes influenced these effects. The potential effects of living with a child with severe learning disabilities are many, but for the child there are benefits in being brought up within the family (Wing, 1985). Not least is the degree of integration and normalisation that can be achieved. It is difficult to measure the success of the move towards community care, but such research that has been undertaken has clearly shown that families and children need easy access to a wide range of services, including practical assistance about managing behavioural problems, financial aid, transport, adaptations to living accommodation, special equipment and respite care on demand (Wing, 1985).

The Future

In this chapter the impact of governmental legislation on care provision for children has been discussed in some depth. The resulting changes have not always, according to much of the literature cited here, resulted in a better-quality service, and many groups of health-care workers are doubtful about how their roles will develop in the future. The changing organisation, management and funding arrangements of many hospital and community services, a different approach to nurse preparation, issues concerned with skill mix as well as new and challenging health-care problems will inevitably mean that we have not yet finished the process of change, nor are we likely to in the foreseeable future. These changes, apart from offering new opportunities for health-care workers, will put pressure on already stretched resources and we will need to become adept at identifying the most efficient and effective ways of providing multidisciplinary care. For example, epidemiological data about HIV infection and AIDS in children tells us that we need to identify ways of caring for whole families who are sick, rather than individuals who traditionally have been segregated according to age, diagnosis and sometimes gender.

Finally, the future is not something over which we have no

power or control. Those of us who are involved in the care of children have the opportunity to make changes which will have an impact as long as good practice is communicated both within professions and between professions.

References

Alder, S. (1991) 'Taking children at their word: pain control in paediatrics', in A. Glasper (ed.) *Child Care: Some Nursing Perspectives*, London: Wolfe Publishing.

Atwell, J. and Gow, M. (1985) 'Paediatric trained district nurses in the community: expensive luxury or economic necessity?' *British Medical Journal*, 291: 227–9.

Bates, T. A. and Broome, M. (1986) 'Preparation of children for hospitalization and surgery: a review of the literature', *Journal of Pediatric Nursing*, 1(4): 30–9.

Battye, J. and Deaken, M. (1979) 'Surveillance reduces baby deaths', *Nursing Mirror*, 148(17): 38–40.

Black, Sir D. (1980) *Inequalities in Health. Report of a Research Working Party*, Chairman: Sir Douglas Black, London: DHSS.

Bowlby, J. (1953) *Child Care and the Growth of Love*, Harmondsworth: Penguin.

British Paediatric Association (1987) Working Party on Paediatric Intensive Care, London: BPA.

Brown, R. (1989) *Individualised Patient Care*, Middlesex: Scutari Press.

Burr, S. (1990) 'Change in the 1990s', *Nursing Standard*, 4(22): 50–1.

Caring for Children in the Health Services Committee (1988) *Parents Staying Overnight with their Children*, London: CCHS Committee.

Carr, J. (1988) '6 weeks to 21 years: a longitudinal study of children with Down's Syndrome and their families', *Journal of Child Psychology and Psychiatry*, 29(4): 407–31.

Clark, J. (1973) *A Family Visitor*, London: RCN.

Clark, J. (1984) 'Mothers' perceptions of health visiting', *Health Visitor*, 57(9): 265–8.

Colliss, V. (1990) 'Pre- and post-operative management', *Paediatric Nursing*, 2(5): 16–17.

Consumers' Association (1980) *Children in Hospital*, London: Consumers' Association.

Consumers' Association (1985) *Children in Hospital*, London: Consumers' Association.

Coulson, D. (1988) 'A proper place for parents', *Nursing Times*, 84(19): 26–8.

Couriel, J. M. and Davies, P. (1988) 'Costs and benefits of a community special care baby service', *British Medical Journal*, 296: 1043–6.

Court, S. D. M. (1976) *Fit for the Future: Report of the Committee on Child Health Services*, Vols I and II, London: HMSO.

Crabbe, G. (1988) 'Public perceptions', *Nursing Times*, 84(42): 70–3.

Craft, M. and Wyatt, N. (1986) 'Effect of visitation upon siblings of hospitalized children', *Maternal–Child Nursing Journal*, 15(1): 47–59.

Currer, C. (1991) 'Understanding the mother's viewpoint: the case of Pathan women in Britain', in S. Wyke and J. Hewison (eds) *Child Health Matters*, Milton Keynes: Open University Press.

Department of Health (1990) *National Health Service and Community Care Act*, London: HMSO.

Department of Health (1989) *Caring for People*, London: HMSO.

Department of Health (1991) *Welfare of Children and Young People in Hospital*, London: HMSO.

Duncan, A., Fernando, M. and Whyte, N. (1986) 'Twilight zone', *Community Outlook*, (May), 14: 16–7.

Eland, J. M. (1988) 'Persistance in pediatric pain research', *Recent Advances in Nursing*, 21: 43–62.

Foster, M. C. and Mayall, B. (1990) 'Health visitors as educators', *Journal of Advanced Nursing*, 15: 286–92.

Fradd, E. (1986) 'It's child's play', *Nursing Times*, 82(41): 40–2.

Fradd, E. (1987) 'Working as a team', *Nursing*, Series 3(24): 900–1.

Gastrell, P. (1986) 'Child health centres – parental and professional views', in A. While (ed.) *Research in Preventive Community Nursing Care*, Chichester: Wiley.

Glasper, A. (1991) 'Parents in the anaesthetic room: a blessing or a curse?' in A. Glasper (ed.) *Child Care: Some Professional Perspectives*, London: Wolfe Publishing.

Glasper, A. Gow, M. and Yerrell, P. (1989) 'A family friend', *Nursing Times*, 85(4): 63–5.

Glen, S. A. (1982) 'Hospital admission through the parent's eyes', *Nursing Times*, 78(31): 1331–3.

Haith, M. M. (1986) 'Sensory and perceptual processes in early infancy', *Journal of Pediatrics*, 109(19): 158–71.

Hall, D. (1987) 'Social and psychological care before and during hospitalisation', *Social Science Medicine*, 25(6): 721–32.

Hall, D. M. B. (1989) *Health for All Children*, London: HMSO.

Harris, P. J. (1988) 'Sometimes pediatric home care doesn't work', *American Journal of Nursing*, 88(6): 851–4.

Hayes, V. E. and Knox, J. E. (1984) 'The experience of stress in parents of children hospitalized with long-term disabilities', *Journal of Advanced Nursing*, 9: 33–41.

Hirose, T. and Veda, R. (1990) 'Long term follow-up study of cerebral palsy children and coping behaviour of parents', *Journal of Advanced Nursing*, 15(7): 762–70.

Holt, H. (1990) 'Southampton's health appraisal pilot study', *Nursing Standard*, 4(16): 26–31.

Husain, M. (1990) 'Parents' attitudes to a child clinic', *Health Visitor*, 63(3): 84.

Jackson, C. (1991) 'Turning back the clock', *Health Visitor*, 64(5): 148–9.

Kitson, A., Atkinson, B. and Ferguson, B. (1987) 'Specialist delivery of care', *Nursing Times*, 83(19): 36–40.

Marriner, J. (1988) 'A children's tour', *Nursing Times*, 84(40): 39–40.

Mattock, C. (1991) 'Stepping off the medical treadmill', *Health Visitor*, 64(5): 154–6.

Mead, D. (1991) 'Nursing management of the injured child in the ward', in D. M. Mead and J. R. Silbert. *The Injured Child*, London: Scutari Press.

Muller, D. J., Harris, P. J., Wattley, L. and Taylor, J. D. (1992) *Nursing Children: Psychology, Research and Practice*, 2nd edn, London: Chapman and Hall.

National Association for the Welfare of Children in Hospital (1990) *Needs and Services of Children in Surgery, Nursing Standard Special Supplement*, 4(24): 14.

Norman, A. (1991) 'Room with a view', *Health Visitor*, 64(4): 103.

Oskala, R. and Merenmies, J. (1989) 'Children's human needs in intensive care', *Intensive Care Nursing*, 5: 155–8.

Perthen, C. (1990) 'Involving the parents', *Nursing*, Series 4(19): 12–16.

Platt, H. (1959) *The Welfare of Children in Hospital: Report of the Committee on Child Health Services*, London: HMSO.

Potrykus, C. (1991) 'Hidden agenda', *Health Visitor*, 64(5): 145.

Powell, J. (1986) 'Study on home visiting of babies in Gosport at high risk of sudden infant death', in A. While (ed.) *Research in Preventive Community Nursing Care*, Chichester: John Wiley.

Prentice, S. (1991) 'What will we find at the market?' *Health Visitor*, 64(1): 9–11.

Radford, P. (1990) 'Physical and emotional care', *Pediatric Nursing*, 2(5): 12–13.

Robertson, J. and Robertson, J. (1989) *Separation and the Very Young*, London: Free Association Books.

Rodin, J. (1983) *Will This Hurt?* London: Scutari Press.

Rukholm, E., Bailey, P. Coutu-Wakulczk, G. and Bailey, W. B. (1991) 'Anxiety levels in relatives of intensive care unit patients', *Journal of Advanced Nursing*, 16: 920–8.

Sefi, S. (1988) 'Health visitors talking to mothers', *Health Visitor*, 61(1): 7–10.

Sherratt, F., Johnson, A. and Holmes, S. (1991) 'Responding to parental concerns at the six-month stage', *Health Visitor*, 64(3): 84–6.

Smallwood, S. (1988) 'Preparing children for surgery', *AORN Journal*, 47(1): 177–85.

Steinberg, D. (1987) *Basic Adolescent Psychiatry*, Oxford: Blackwell Scientific Publications.

Taylor, J. (1991) 'Health behaviour and beliefs', *Health Visitor*, 61(7): 223–4.

Vine, P. (1991) 'Ninety-nine and counting', *Health Visitor*, 64(5): 150–1.

Wailes, J. (1983) 'Non-accidental injury', *Nursing Mirror*, 157(16): 20–2.

Watson, E. (1991) '"Appropriate" use of child health services in East London: ethnic similarities and differences', in S. Wyke and J. Hewison (eds) *Child Health Matters*, Milton Keynes: Open University Press.

Weatherley, D. (1988) 'A survey of clients' views in one health visitor's caseload', *Health Visitor*, 61(5): 137–8.

Weller, B. (1980) *Helping Sick Children Play*, London: Baillière Tindall.

Whiting, M. (1989) 'Home truths', *Nursing Times*, 85(14): 74–5.

Willcox, A. (1990) 'Children in the surgery practice', *Nurse*, 3(2): 92–3, 96.

Wing, K. (1985) 'Services for severely retarded children and adolescents', in M. Rutter and L. Hersov. (eds) *Child and Adolescent Psychiatry*, 2nd edn, Oxford: Blackwell Scientific Publications.

PART 4

CONCLUSIONS

12

A FUTURE FOR CHILD-CARE NURSING?

Bruce Lindsay
Norfolk College of Nursing and Midwifery

The preceding chapters have focused on a wide range of issues
affecting the health care of children. While each chapter's
focus is different, each discussion takes account of issues which
are the subject of focus elsewhere. This approach by the individual authors was not deliberate. However, its occurrence
throughout the book emphasises one element of importance
for the continued development of effective child health care:
integration of health-care services, health-care professionals,
families and children. This idea of integration is one of the
themes which appears consistently across the individual
chapters.

A second theme is to be found with equal consistency: the
theme of change. In Part 1 changes to and within society are
shown to have major effects on children. Part 2 identifies four
areas of change in the influences on and approaches to child
health care in the 1990s. The contributors to Part 3, focusing
on ways forward, are themselves asking for change – to
current practice or to existing perceptions.

The third major theme can also be found in many of the earlier discussions: the theme of choice. What choices are made
about child health care? Who makes those choices? What
freedom of choice is available to the child-care nurse, the child
or the family? How should these choices best be exercised?
What influences do these choices have on the effectiveness of
child health care?

These three themes have major implications for children's
health care and, therefore, for child-care nurses. They affect
the care which is given, the children and families who receive

care and the ways in which we work as individuals and as multi-disciplinary team members. They influence the ways in which child-care nurses are prepared and the ways in which they can develop and improve as practitioners. They can be seen as challenges or threats, as barriers or as opportunities. They cannot, however, simply be ignored.

Integrating Care

The notion of an integrated approach to child health care is becoming central to government ideas regarding this service. The provision of a 'seamless web of care' (Department of Health, 1991) is seen as the ideal. However, it is interesting to note the differing amounts and types of integration to which the contributors refer. First, the integration of child health services and the professionals who work within them. Secondly, integration on a more microscopic level within a defined framework of care: a framework which itself affects the degree of integration which is seen as desirable. Thirdly, integration of knowledge and understanding into nursing practice.

Perhaps the single most important type of integration considered here is the integration of the child into the decision-making process. How far can, or should, an individual child be allowed to participate in decisions affecting care and treatment? How ready are child-care nurses to implement care based in part, or even wholly, on the decisions of the child? Will we do so even when those decisions contradict those of the parents or the health professionals? These questions may well be answered positively by most child-care nurses in certain circumstances. But how vital must such decisions become before most of us say 'No, those decisions are no longer for the child to take'?

The Challenge of Change

Health care in contemporary Britain continues to go through change after change in the way services are provided, in the way they are financed, in the way they are managed. The ways in which nurses and other health professionals are prepared are also changing, as are the public's expectations of them. The degree of involvement of children and their families in decisions about care is changing. The influences upon our health are changing, as are the ways in which these influences act and the social structures in which they act and must be responded to.

Many changes to the types of family structure have occurred

in the last few hundred years, leading to changes in our understanding of 'the family' and our expectations of its role and
function. Changes to society's expectations of and for children
are central to the development of children's rights and of
children's places within power relationships.

Without technological change, the medical and nursing care
now available within, for example, neonatal units would not be
possible. However, such units do exist, and this change in care
provision brings with it a complete alteration in our expectations for the very premature or low birth weight baby.
Technological change has also altered, and continues to alter,
the role of the media as an influence on development. A further
aspect of change is particularly clear in this context: rapid
change keeps ahead of our responses to it.

The Right to Choose

The first version of this theme looks at who chooses; the second
considers the influences (including constraints) upon choice; the
third focuses on ways in which choices can be informed so that
they can be made as effectively as possible.

This concept of choice, of decision making, pervades all levels
of child health care. On a global scale, decisions are taken which
may affect the rights of the child or the route along which developments in care may take place. On a local level choices will
influence the availability of child health services and hence the
availability of choices which children and families have regarding health care. On a micro-level the availability or non-
availability of choice will have major effects on the success or
failure of individual health-care episodes.

It is also important to understand who makes these choices
about the health care of children: international organisations,
such as the United Nations or World Health Organisation;
national and local governments; health service managers at regional and local levels; fund-holding general practices; medical
consultants, senior nurses and senior members of other health
professions; individual health visitors, nurses, parents or carers;
and individual children. Each has a degree of choice, with its
importance for individual cases varying with the circumstances.

Influences on choice are many and varied. Choices can be
influenced by the frameworks within which care takes place. An
approach to care which excludes the aim of caring for the child
and family as a unit – the old 'task allocation' model, for
example – is likely to deny many opportunities for choice on the

part of the family. Indeed, it is also likely to exert a negative influence on the choices available to individual nurses with regard to their care, with its tendency to centralise the control of care to a single 'team leader'. Another model, such as the 'partnership' approach (Casey, 1988), exerts a more positive influence, enabling much greater opportunities for choice for individual staff as well as for children and families.

So how can child-care nurses best inform their choices about child health? By the effective use of research and an expansion of research with a specific child health focus, helping to increase knowledge and understanding. By a greater understanding of the child, and the child's beliefs and wishes, whether in connection with a choice of TV programme or a choice of health-care treatment. Children's nurses should, in most cases, have access to many sources of information which can help in making our choices. For children and parents such access may be much more restricted and making informed choices becomes more difficult.

Integration, Change and Choice

Together, these three themes represent major challenges for children's nursing. Changes to health-care needs and to the provision of health services mean that children's nurses must make choices about how they themselves will change to function effectively in the new (and still changing) health-care environment. As the increasing integration of child health-care services is favoured in the 1990s, child-care nurses need to change aspects of their practice and preparation in order to continue to hold a vital and unique role. But what makes child-care nursing unique?

Child-care Nursing: Unique within Nursing?

Whether or not nursing is a unique activity within health care, can the nursing care of children be seen as a unique area of nursing practice? Foster (1989) states that 'the goal of pediatric nursing is to promote the healthy maturation of the child/adolescent as a physical, intellectual, and emotional-social being within the context of the family and the community'. She goes on to claim that it is this promotion of healthy maturation which makes the nursing care of children and adolescents unique. This can be said to be a uniqueness of both action (the promotion of healthy maturation) and knowledge (of, for example, development and the effects of illness upon it).

Other nurses may disagree with the claim to uniqueness of action. Members of other professional groups may disagree with the claim to uniqueness of knowledge: child-care nurses make use of knowledge gained from a wide range of sources but as yet have little claim to any body of knowledge which they have developed independently. However, child-care nurses use their knowledge to act in particular ways for the benefit of an identified client group (children and families) with health-related needs. While other nurses do care for children and families, with the goal of healthy maturation in mind, they do so without the specialist knowledge of the child-care nurse. Other professionals may have similar knowledge to apply to their care of children, but it is used in different ways to meet different needs.

So the uniqueness of child-care nursing can be seen as resulting from a combination of the ways in which knowledge is put into action and the goals which this action attempts to achieve. But this uniqueness does not in itself make child-care nursing an indispensable element of health care. We must ensure that the goals we set are worth achieving and are viewed as such by those for whom we work. We must also ensure that our knowledge and our abilities in practice are sufficient to enable us to achieve the goals. Child-care nurses cannot afford to stand still, but must continue to evaluate and develop the role.

The Way Ahead?

So what is the way ahead for child-care nursing? Is there a single path, or should we be using many routes towards our goal of improved children's nursing care? Do we look inside or outside the profession for indicators of how the profession should develop? Does the future lie in an expansion of an autonomous role for the children's nurse or in greater integration with other health professionals?

The answers to these questions will surely lie in a single imperative for child-care nursing: developing the service to best meet the nursing needs of children and families. However, a major national report suggests that this development still has some way to go.

Hospital services for children: an independent view

In early 1993, as this chapter was nearing completion, the Audit Commission published its report *'Children First: a Study of*

Hospital Services'. This detailed report identifies and supports six principles for the care of children in hospital, going on to establish the extent to which British hospital services are failing to achieve them and suggesting ways in which improvements can be made.

The Commission's report is supportive of many of the ideas expressed by the contributors to this book. It clearly sees children as having different health-care needs from those of adults. It recognises that children's nurses need specialist preparation to enable them to develop the special skills which are necessary for the successful nursing care of children and their families. It emphasises the importance of health-care settings dedicated to children, and the importance of a well-developed community nursing service for children. But it also provides evidence to show that in many ways the Health Service continues to fail in its provision of children's health care.

The six principles, as the Audit Commission itself notes, 'are not new and are (already) accepted by many of the national organisations involved'. They are:

- the principle of child and family-centred care;
- the need for specially skilled staff (from all disciplines, not solely nursing);
- separate facilities for children (in specialist departments such as accident and emergency, as well as wards);
- effective treatments (the report suggests that in some cases children receive unnecessary, ineffective treatments);
- appropriate hospitalisation (where 'there is a therapeutic advantage to the child over care at home');
- strategic commissioning (defined as 'having a clear strategy based on needs and ensuring that it is effectively and efficiently implemented').

The child-care nurse is crucial for all of these principles, and the fact that the Audit Commission finds none of the principles being successfully achieved nationally should therefore be of great concern to us.

Our responses to the shortcomings noted in the report need to be identified on two basic levels. Where the shortcomings are viewed as resulting from a failure of management strategies, whether at local, regional or national level, then we as individuals, or through organisations, need to exert influence to ensure that strategies become more favourable towards children. Examples given by the Audit Commission include the lack of qualified children's nurses, the lack of separate facilities and ineffective treatment (the report cites the specific example of children with glue ear).

Other criticisms are much more specifically directed at nurses. The lack of children's nurses on duty on children's wards during particular shifts, for example, when compared to the Department of Health standard of at least two qualified children's nurses on duty twenty-four hours a day (Department of Health, 1991) is not solely the result of an overall lack of suitably qualified nurses, according to the report. Its authors also suggest that in some cases at least it is the result of ward management which 'did not even consider the standard as an issue in rostering'.

Perhaps most important of all is the principle of child and family-centred care. This principle is a cornerstone of contemporary child-care nursing, and yet the Commission reports regarding this principle that

> The root problem identified in the Audit Commission study is that *clinicians, managers and other staff do not give sufficient attention to the needs of children and their families*. It is manifest in a lack of written policies, management focus and poor communication between staff and parents.
>
> (Audit Commission, 1993: 10; their emphasis)

This criticism is not levelled solely, or even primarily, at nurses. But it is supported by examples of bad practice in areas where nurses have a major responsibility, particularly regarding communication with children and parents, and the confusion of parents regarding their role in caring for their hospitalised children.

The way in which children's nurses respond to these findings will be crucial for the future. It is certainly possible to identify examples of good practice in wards and departments across the country with which to counter the report's criticisms. But it is also important to accept that these criticisms are valid and that bad practice does occur. We need to be willing to accept that difficulties exist, and to deal with them constructively and publicly. Where this means that changes to practice or role are needed, then such changes should be driven from within the specialism, and should be supported by research evidence. This may help to ensure that our criticisms of others will be listened to with respect and acted upon as being those of a truly knowledgeable and professional group.

In recent decades major changes to children's health care have seen equally major changes to the role of the children's nurse. One example is the move towards parental involvement in hospital-based care. The move from limited parental access to hospitalised children to the provision of residential accommodation for parents brought with it the change in the role of the children's nurse from a 'private' role, with nursing care carried out in the absence of parents, to a much more public one, with nursing care given under almost constant supervision by parents.

As parents became participants in care, rather than simply observers, the focus of the role changed still further. Nurses and parents became integrated into a caring team, a partnership. However, although parents continue to take primary responsibility for the vast majority of the care of sick children at home, hospital-based partnerships continue to see the professionals as the 'senior partners' in most instances, retaining responsibility for 'nursing' care.

Further moves, which are still continuing, create yet more changes in the nurse's role. The move from parental involvement in care to a situation where parents accept almost total responsibility for the care of their hospitalised child in a 'care by parents unit' (Cleary, 1992) results in the child-care nurse needing the skills of teaching and facilitation in order to function effectively. In such units, which are well-established in the United States although less so in the United Kingdom, nurses are there to offer education and support to the parents, and to take over from them in the giving of care only when necessary (Evans, 1991). Such a development requires major changes in the preparation of children's nurses and in the definition of their role. However, while Glasper (1990) notes that many children's units are making genuine and successful attempts at involving parents, he also emphasises that 'the concept of family centred care has yet to gain universal approval'. The time when the right of the parents to continue to act as primary caregivers for the hospitalised child, rather than merely having the right to be present throughout the child's stay, is accepted universally appears still to be some time away.

The reluctance of many child-care nurses to facilitate the expansion of parental responsibility into more technical, 'professional' and decision-making aspects of care is perhaps understandable. However, this expansion should instead be seen as positive for families, children and child-care nurses alike. Indeed, it would seem to be vital for the development of community-centred child-care nursing that parental responsibility expands into areas of care previously viewed as the domain of the hospital-based nurse. Certainly, if child-care nurses are confident enough of their own role and abilities to be able to support families in the continuation of care for their children, wherever that care takes place, then such a move should strengthen the professionalism of child-care nursing rather than threaten it. However, it is vital for the success of this move that parental responsibility for nursing care is seen as a *right* and not as an obligation. Devolution of care must not be undertaken to the point where the parents are unable or unwilling to carry it out.

Planning for the Future

Child-care nursing has a future, albeit an uncertain one as the climate of change continues to affect all areas of health care. The following 'five-point plan' identifies a series of elements which are of particular importance in ensuring that this future is one which enhances child and family care, and the role of child-care nursing within it.

1 Overt recognition by child-care nurses of the primacy of the child.
2 Continued integration of children and their families in decisions about children's care.
3 Increased devolution of direct care to family members (within the limits of their wishes and abilities), and to community settings.
4 Recognition of the effects of change and the need to act *proactively* to control these effects.
5 More involvement in influencing decisions about child health policy and practice, in particular by the establishment of a body of nursing research.

None of these elements is itself new. However, taken together they can enable children's nurses, individually or collectively, to focus on the future in a way which will encourage the development of the specialism as one with increasing importance for the health care of children.

Overt recognition of the primacy of the child in all aspects of our work simply encourages the public presentation of a belief which all child-care nurses should hold privately. Such a public presentation helps to ensure that people outside the specialism can judge its actions against this agreed view: it does not require that all child-care nurses necessarily agree on the best way to ensure this primacy.

One way in which contemporary child-care nurses believe the primacy of the child can be achieved is reflected in the second and third elements of the plan. Further integration of children and families into the decision making process, coupled with more devolution of direct care to family members and home settings, gives them more power and control with regard to the management of care. It has also been argued that such moves should be seen as indicators of a strong confidence on the part of child-care nursing: as signs of a specialism secure in its unique position in child health care.

Maintaining this unique position requires the fourth element: being proactive in recognising and dealing with the effects of change. Achieving this proactive role requires element five, involvement in the formulation of policy and the establishment of a body of nursing research.

Two recent publications offer children's nurses, both individually and collectively, the opportunity to advance the achievement of this plan and to establish themselves as at the forefront of nursing practice. The report 'A Vision for the Future' (Department of Health, 1993a) sets out a series of targets for the key areas of quality, accountability, clinical leadership, purchasing and education, and identifies the 1989 Children Act as a crucial policy initiative. Many of the areas of importance, such as individualised care or 'users involvement in care' are areas which children's nurses have been involved with for many years. The recognition of their importance gives an ideal opportunity for the specialism to demonstrate its well-established abilities in these areas.

The 'Report of the Taskforce on the Strategy for Research in Nursing, Midwifery and Health Visiting' (Department of Health, 1993b) establishes a total of thirty-seven recommendations for the development of research. Many of these offer opportunities for child-care nurses to develop research skills or to take up project funding. At the time of writing no decision has yet been taken by the government on whether or not to act on these recommendations, but we must be ready to take advantage of any government action whenever it takes place. It may be the specialism's best chance for many years to establish a research base of its own with which to advance child-care nursing practice.

Conclusion

Children's nursing is not alone in facing an uncertain future. The latter part of the twentieth century has seen a dramatic reappraisal of health-care provision throughout the world: as a response to new threats such as AIDS; as a result of shifts in government thinking about the means of provision, shown particularly vividly in the changes to Britain's Health Service; or as part of an overall change in society's attitude to health and health care, reflected in the growth in complementary therapies in Western nations. Nurses in all specialities have seen major changes to the ways in which they are prepared, to the service they are able to provide and to their relationship with other health professionals and with their patients and clients.

Children's nursing does, however, have its own particular perspectives on these uncertainties which stem from its beliefs about its role in the health care of children, If, as we believe, children's nursing is truly a unique and vital element in child health care, then the ways in which it will develop to meet the challenges of the future will be vitally important not only for its expansion as a specialism but also for the future well-being of the world's children.

References

Audit Commission (1993) *Children First: a Study of Hospital Services*, London: HMSO.

Casey, A. (1988) 'A partnership with child and family', *Senior Nurse*, 8(4): 8.

Cleary, J. (1992) *Caring for Children in Hospital*, London: Scutari Press.

Department of Health (1991) *Welfare of Children and Young People in Hospital*, London: HMSO.

Department of Health (1993a) *A Vision for the Future*, London: HMSO.

Department of Health (1993b) *Report of the Taskforce on the Strategy for Research in Nursing, Midwifery and Health Visiting*, London: HMSO.

Evans, M. (1991) 'Caring by parents', in A. Glasper (ed.) *Child Care: Some Nursing Perspectives*, London: Wolfe Publishing Ltd.

Foster, R. L. R. (1989) 'Perspectives on the nursing care of children and adolescents', in R. L. R. Foster, M. M. Hunsberger and J. J. T. Anderson (eds) *Family-centered Nursing Care of Children*, Philadelphia: W. B. Saunders.

Glasper, A. (1990) 'Emancipation of parents', *Nursing Standard*, 4(22): 55.

INDEX